# IN TUNE

## EXERCISES TO IMPROVE A MUSICIAN'S PERFORMANCE AND QUALITY OF LIFE

Jaume Rosset i Llobet

Sílvia Fàbregas i Molas

**TRANSLATED AND LOCALIZED**

Annie Bosler, DMA and Dylan Skye Hart, MM

This publication contains the opinions of its authors. The information, exercises, and advice contained in this book are not intended as a substitute for working with a healthcare professional. The publisher and authors are not responsible for any adverse effects or consequences resulting from the use of the materials in this book. Consult your healthcare professional before starting a new exercise routine or program.

The authors, Jaume Rosset i Llobet and Sílvia Fàbregas i Molas, are exclusive owners of the copyright to *A tono: Ejercicios para mejorar el rendimiento del músico*, the underlying Spanish language version of this work. Silver Bells Music, Inc. is the exclusive copyright owner of *In Tune: Exercises to Improve a Musician's Performance and Quality of Life*, the English language translation, and all supplemental material.

*A tono: Ejercicios para mejorar el rendimiento del músico* ©2005 Jaume Rosset i Llobet and Sílvia Fàbregas i Molas. English language translation: *In Tune: Exercises to Improve a Musician's Performance and Quality of Life* and all supplemental material ©2023 Silver Bells Music, Inc. All rights reserved.

This book or any portion thereof may not be reproduced or used in any manner whatsoever without the express written permission of the publisher except for the use of brief quotations in a book review.

Published by Silver Bells Music, Inc.

ISBN 978-0-578-73946-5
ISBN (e-book) 978-0-578-73947-2

Interior artwork: Jaume Rosset i Llobet
Book layout design: Terese Harris and *the*BookDesigners
Book cover design: *the*BookDesigners

Printed in the United States of America
First English Printing, 2023

## SPECIAL THANK YOU:

Mark Adams, Erin Armstrong, Terese Harris, Mika Judge, Marilyn Bone Kloss, and Jacqueline Petito

# TABLE OF CONTENTS

**Foreword** . . . . . . . . . . . . . . . . . . . . . . . . . . . . . . . . . . . . . . . . . . . . *vii*

**Prologue** . . . . . . . . . . . . . . . . . . . . . . . . . . . . . . . . . . . . . . . . . . . . *ix*

**1: Introduction** . . . . . . . . . . . . . . . . . . . . . . . . . . . . . . . . . . . . . . . 1

**2: Basic Concepts** . . . . . . . . . . . . . . . . . . . . . . . . . . . . . . . . . . . . . 5
    **Flexibility Exercises** . . . . . . . . . . . . . . . . . . . . . . . . . . . . . . . . . 7
    **Stretching Exercises** . . . . . . . . . . . . . . . . . . . . . . . . . . . . . . . 13
    **Toning Exercises** . . . . . . . . . . . . . . . . . . . . . . . . . . . . . . . . . . 19
    **Warming up and Cooling down** . . . . . . . . . . . . . . . . . . . . . . . 24

**3: Exercises by Region of the Body** . . . . . . . . . . . . . . . . . . . . . . 27
    **Hand** . . . . . . . . . . . . . . . . . . . . . . . . . . . . . . . . . . . . . . . . . . . . 29
    **Forearm** . . . . . . . . . . . . . . . . . . . . . . . . . . . . . . . . . . . . . . . . . 38
    **Arm, Shoulder, and Chest** . . . . . . . . . . . . . . . . . . . . . . . . . . . 45
    **Neck and Dorsal Region of the Back** . . . . . . . . . . . . . . . . . . . 57
    **Lumbar and Abdominals** . . . . . . . . . . . . . . . . . . . . . . . . . . . 64
    **Thigh and Leg** . . . . . . . . . . . . . . . . . . . . . . . . . . . . . . . . . . . . 73
    **Face** . . . . . . . . . . . . . . . . . . . . . . . . . . . . . . . . . . . . . . . . . . . . 79

**4: Exercises by Instrument** . . . . . . . . . . . . . . . . . . . . . . . . . . . . 87
    **Wind, Front** . . . . . . . . . . . . . . . . . . . . . . . . . . . . . . . . . . . . . 96
    **Small Wind, Front** . . . . . . . . . . . . . . . . . . . . . . . . . . . . . . . .106
    **Wind, Side** . . . . . . . . . . . . . . . . . . . . . . . . . . . . . . . . . . . . . .114
    **Wind, Lateral** . . . . . . . . . . . . . . . . . . . . . . . . . . . . . . . . . . . .123
    **Bowed String, Front** . . . . . . . . . . . . . . . . . . . . . . . . . . . . . .132
    **Large Bowed String** . . . . . . . . . . . . . . . . . . . . . . . . . . . . . .140
    **Bowed String, Shoulder** . . . . . . . . . . . . . . . . . . . . . . . . . . .149
    **Plucked String** . . . . . . . . . . . . . . . . . . . . . . . . . . . . . . . . . . .157

| | |
|---|---|
| Plucked String, Harp | 166 |
| Percussion | 175 |
| Percussion, Drum Set | 183 |
| Keyboard | 192 |
| Keyboard with Hands and Feet | 200 |
| Brass | 209 |
| Brass, Lateral | 218 |

**5: Staying Healthy and Fit** . . . . . . . . . . . . . . . . . . . . . . . . . . . . . . . 227

**6: Exercises for Special Situations** . . . . . . . . . . . . . . . . . . . . . . . . 245

**7: Exercises that are Advised Against** . . . . . . . . . . . . . . . . . . . . . . 251

**Appendices**

| | |
|---|---|
| Glossary of Muscles | 257 |
| Glossary of Terms | 289 |

**Index** . . . . . . . . . . . . . . . . . . . . . . . . . . . . . . . . . . . . . . . . . . . . . . . 301

# FOREWORD

As the daughter of a collegiate football and track star, I learned at a young age the importance of warming up, stretching, strength training, and cooling down. I grew up with a tennis racquet in one hand and a French horn in the other. I was constantly running off a tennis court to go to orchestra rehearsal or a music lesson. As a result, I figured out early in my career that musicians, whether they realize it or not, are athletes. Musicians and athletes both spend hours practicing their craft. The strains and stresses on their bodies due to repetitive motion are similar. However, most musicians are not as diligent as athletes about taking care of their bodies.

In addition, musicians have been slower than athletes to adopt a culture of openness about pain or injury. While sports medicine was a term coined in 1928, the term music medicine was not established until 1982. When athletes are hurt, they admit it and get help. When musicians experience pain or become injured, they often do not feel comfortable talking about it and hide it from colleagues, hoping things will heal on their own. This reluctance to admit to pain or injury seems to span all genres and types of musicians. It is time to change this paradigm for the sake of musicians everywhere.

I first came across the work of Dr. Jaume Rosset i Llobet in 2009 on a trip to Australia. In the Queensland Conservatorium gift shop, I found the book that he wrote with George Odam, *The Musician's Body: a maintenance manual for peak performance*. I read it cover-to-cover and was beyond excited to find someone that not only understood anatomy and physiology, but took the world of sports and merged it into the land of music.

I later came across another book, *A tono: ejercicios para mejorar el rendimiento del músico*. Although this book was in Spanish, Dr. Rosset put into words and pictures what

## FOREWORD

I had understood many years earlier: musicians can use calisthenics, stretching, work outs, and cross training to maintain their bodies just like athletes do.

This translation project was a massive undertaking. Thank you to Dr. Rosset for his infinite patience and to Hollywood studio musician Dylan Skye Hart, who endeavored on this several thousand hour journey with me. It would not have been possible without them. I have used this work countless times in my teaching, including in a TEDx lecture called *Elissa's Song: The Power of Exercising Your Face*. It is my hope that this book provides a gateway for more communication about wellness within the music community.

**Annie Bosler, DMA**
Professional French horn player
Embouchure and face anatomy specialist
www.anniebosler.com
Silver Bells Music, Inc.

# PROLOGUE

Since ancient times, the people of Egypt, Greece, and India have used sound frequencies to heighten awareness and to rejuvenate the body and spirit. When these sound frequencies were ordered harmonically, becoming music, they would restore balance and release stress, offsetting the negative patterns that accumulated in the energy field.

However, this application of sound as a therapeutic property of music does not relieve or prevent many musicians from suffering various kinds of medical problems related to their craft.

On behalf of these musicians, I want to introduce this magnificent work that attempts to create an awareness of the effort involved in the repetitive motions and physical consequences of energy expenditure among musicians.

This book gives practical exercises that prepare musicians to perform their best, avoid injury, and reestablish well-being. Also included are facts and statistics that are useful for all kinds of musicians, not just for those who play daily in large ensembles.

I have always admired the special relationship that dancers have with their bodies. Teachers and students of dance share knowledge about physical care, injury prevention, and body maintenance that they have acquired since the beginning of their artistic training.

By contrast, most musicians know almost nothing about the physical mechanics of the body and how it relates to playing, how to utilize the body to get the best results without injury, and the proper position of the body in relation to individual instruments.

# PROLOGUE

I reiterate my gratitude to this unique and significant study of the consequences, derivations, and solutions to the practice of a vocation that inevitably becomes a profession: music.

There are scholars who say: "We are all musical." Intrinsic to human nature, each person has the gift of music within themselves. "Music and rhythm are, of course, life."

This book will aid musicians to replenish and improve their outlook and condition, in the same way that music heightens awareness and rejuvenates the body and spirit.

I do not want to take any more time away from your reading and digesting this book that addresses a very important topic for artists and performers: injury prevention and physical development.

I am sure that this profound book of research will help musicians maintain high spirits, enjoy their performances, and sustain their well-being.

**Luis Cobos**
Musician
*President of the Spanish Society of Artists*

# Chapter One

# INTRODUCTION

# IN TUNE

Musical accomplishment is founded on the mastery of close to perfect instrumental technique. Not in vain, the refinement of physical movement is one of the fundamental goals of the musician both as a student and as a professional.

Although it has been proven that this refinement can be achieved, at least in part, by mental work, learning is mostly based on repetition of the movements required for playing an instrument. This repetition, if sufficient and performed under discerning conditions, leads to the automation of the movement, allowing the musician to achieve greater nuance and speed of execution. Unfortunately, most musicians base this process on hours of repetition each day without long breaks or significant rest.

Although a part of what you learn becomes engraved forever, many of the more complex actions are far from permanent. To retain these, it is imperative that once the desired degree of refinement is reached, you continue to practice.

This goes to illustrate that from the beginning until the end of your career, you must always devote many hours on the repetition of movements and gestures required for playing your instrument.

Although it is undeniable that coordinated movements occur through the contraction and relaxation of multiple muscles, musicianS are generally not consciously aware that the movements they are making require an expenditure of energy and involve physical consequences that are often subtle.

In the musician's case, it is often found that the act of playing an instrument is not commonly related to the physiological changes that are usually associated with physical exertion: acceleration of the heart and respiratory system, sweating, feeling of exhaustion and stiffness, etc. This is probably why there is a lack of awareness that performing is a strenuous exercise. Certainly, many musicians have not received training that incorporates education about the body and how it works. Furthermore, should the need for bodily care or rehabilitation arise, musicians do not possess the appropriate tools for this to be accomplished.

# CHAPTER ONE

## INTRODUCTION

Undesired consequences can result from repeating the same gesture multiple times under adverse conditions and without adequate consideration from the physical point of view. Health studies of musicians conducted in various countries have found that a high percentage of musicians (higher than 75%) end up having physical ailments at some point in their life that affect their musical progression and professional career.

The exercises and activities that can help counterbalance these problems in musicians do not necessarily follow the same principles that govern the world of sports. It is often thought that building muscle at the gym, using springs to strengthen hands, or a long swim in a pool every week will offset the stresses of playing a musical instrument. However, this is not the case.

A musician's muscles should combine agility, resistance, elasticity, and strength. These attributes must be worked on in a balanced way and, moreover, without overburdening or adding extra risk to the structures or areas that are already vulnerable.

As a general rule, musicians need exercises that yield the most benefit when playing their instrument while simultaneously protecting them from the likelihood of injury and contributing to restoring the body. In order to do this, musicians must counteract the created tension and rebalance the areas that were worked both when playing and when exercising.

Do not make the mistake of thinking that only musicians who have been injured or professionals who play many hours a day need to do these exercises. Obviously, for these groups of musicians (injured and professionals), the exercises that follow will be especially useful if incorporated into a daily routine. However, these routines can also be beneficial for any category of musician including students in their first years of instrumental training, amateurs who play sporadically, symphony orchestra players, and recording artists, as well as those who play rock, folk, or pop music.

For more information, download **Musician's First Aid**, a free app available on Android and iOS.

## THIS BOOK CONTAINS...

This is a manual for musicians consisting primarily of exercises. In order for the instrumentalist to fully incorporate these exercises into their practice routine, it is essential to understand the usefulness of the exercises and why they have been chosen.

This book includes the following chapters:

**Basic Concepts**. Explains each type of exercise, for whom they are intended, and how they can be done.

**Exercises by Region of the Body.** Musicians will learn exercises to suit their needs. The exercises are grouped by region of the body. Each region includes exercises for flexibility (improving joint mobility and muscle elasticity), stretching (lengthening the muscles and reducing tension), and toning (enhancing strength and muscle endurance). Musicians must take into account the reasons and instructions provided for each of the exercises described so as to maximize results and avoid injury.

**Exercises by Instrument.** Recommended routines for individual instruments are grouped by similar playing posture. This includes a pre-playing routine (warm-up) and a post-playing routine (cool-down). These routines are specially designed to address the demands and strains made on the body by each instrument.

**Staying Healthy and Fit.** A general exercise program is proposed for those musicians who wish to work comprehensively on the whole body to improve their physical condition both on their instrument and in their daily lives.

In *Exercises by Instrument* and *Staying Healthy and Fit*, two versions have been designed: Essential, a basic version which includes exercises necessary for maintaining a desirable physical condition, and Complete, a full version for those who have more time and want to ensure peak fitness and improved physical performance.

**Exercises for Special Situations.** Ideas are included for how you can modify the exercises in this book so that they can be done in less than ideal conditions. An example of this would be using the adapted exercises while you are on stage during a rehearsal.

**Exercises that are Advised Against.** Although certain exercises may be perfectly fine in other contexts or activities, this chapter contains a list of exercises that are not advised for any musician and could be harmful. Justifications are included as to why each exercise on this list is not advised.

## AN APPENDIX IS INCLUDED WITH THE FOLLOWING GLOSSARIES:

**Glossary of Muscles.** The main muscles used by musicians are described in this section. This is not a treatise on anatomy. Rather, it is a basic overview of the elements that allow musicians to play, resulting in a better understanding of how the muscles do and do not work. For easy reference, these muscle names appear in italics as they are mentioned throughout the book, followed by a number referencing the order in which the word appears in the glossary.

**Glossary of Terms.** This section describes and illustrates medical concepts used in this book. The terms appear in italics throughout the book to let the reader know which terms can be found in the glossary.

Chapter Two

# BASIC CONCEPTS

As already mentioned, the presence of physical problems in musician originate essentially from inadequate understanding of the body and high expectations of fine movement that is involved in playing an instrument. Such demands are determined by incessant, often obsessive, repetition of movements in improper ergonomic positions under excessive stress and adverse conditions. The tension and poor posture can cause *muscle contractions* (spasms) and loss of muscular elasticity. These repetitive motions and asymmetrical gestures lead to imbalances in the muscles. An imbalanced, inelastic, and stiff muscle will not only worsen performance but increase susceptibility to injury.

It has been determined that flexibility, stretching, and toning exercises can contribute to the prevention and/or restoration of damaged areas. These kinds of exercises are easy to understand and follow. They are perfectly suited to the needs and movement requirements of musicians. Also, these exercises are rarely harmful, even if misunderstood and/or poorly performed.

# CHAPTER TWO — BASIC CONCEPTS

# FLEXIBILITY EXERCISES

### Definition

Flexibility is being able to perform movements throughout your full range and harness the potential strength of efficient joint movement.

Joint mobility, muscle elasticity, and other factors including heredity, climate, fatigue, and most importantly age determine overall flexibility. As you age, flexibility decreases, especially if you do not cultivate it.

Flexibility exercises are intended to preserve and improve your range of motion. Even some stretching exercises, which will be mentioned later, can be considered flexibility exercises.

A simple example would be pianists who want to warm up their finger agility. These pianists would perform a flexibility exercise by alternating finger movements, in all directions, which involves the joints and muscles in the finger area. Here you can see examples of *finger flexion-extension* (bend and straighten) and abduction-adduction (separate and together) which allows for the proper preparation of a pianist's hands.

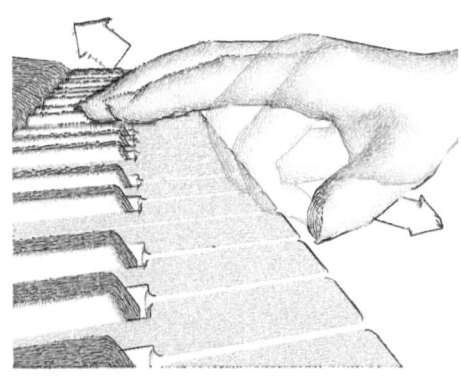

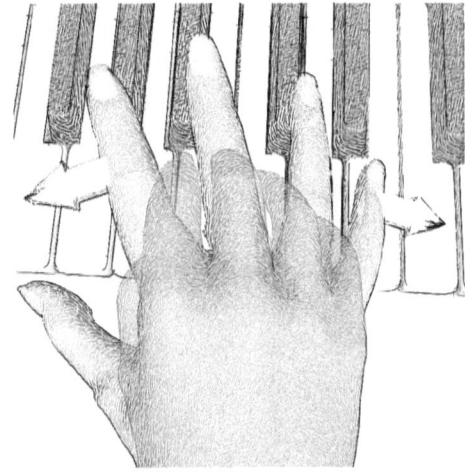

*To make the hand more flexible before playing, it is recommended to do several exercises such as those shown in the figures. These exercises will warm the muscles, improve fluidity of joint movement, and increase blood flow to the muscles and tendons.*

## Purpose:

Flexibility is a physical quality that is essential for achieving correct and efficient execution of movement. These exercises seek to maintain fluid, free-working joint mobility as well as to promote efficient muscle coordination. The exercises are also intended to pursue a degree of elasticity and proper muscle tone for playing.

As a general concept, in addition to assisting in maintaining flexibility and preparation of the muscles for stretching, they are a good progression for passing salubriously from rest to activity.

## Who Can Do This?

All musicians should work regularly on flexibility. Furthermore, since it is a quality that is lost with the passage of time, this work should be more intense the older one gets. However, while it is true that children have ample elasticity and mobility, it would be advisable to introduce these activities at an early age to stimulate the body so as not to have any regressions in flexibility.

Although these are light exercises and are in principle suitable for all musicians, if you have an injury, seek medical advice (preferably from a professional who has experience working with musicians) to see if any of the exercises could be harmful.

## When and Where?

Although flexibility exercises can be done whenever and wherever you want, at minimum, they should be performed before playing your instrument.

Anytime you notice any area of the body beginning to stiffen due to repetitive activity, posture, or stress, flexibility exercises can restore mobility and elasticity as well as avoid future problems.

## Equipment:

You do not need any special equipment or clothing; however, a relaxed atmosphere, pleasant temperature, and comfortable loose clothing facilitate the implementation.

For floor exercises, it is better, although not essential, to have a towel, blanket, or mat for comfort.

## How to:

The basic principle is to perform smooth and slow movements (taking several seconds for each motion) without stressing or forcing any bodily structure. Therefore, the

# CHAPTER TWO — BASIC CONCEPTS

recommended process is to repeat a movement (usually between 10 and 15 times), always returning to the starting point without halting or pausing between repetitions.

For added benefit, slightly change the position of any of the joints that are directly or indirectly related to the movement of the exercise. For example, in the exercise *1-Finger mobility* (page 29), the wrist can be placed in different degrees of *extension* or *flexion*, the fingers can be bent or straightened, the palm of the hand can be facing up or down, etc. It is advisable to work the areas that will experience intense activity, require a high degree of mobility, or remain in a sustained position while playing.

Although each exercise has a specific posture to which you must adhere for correct execution, some general rules apply to all exercises contained herein. These rules also serve for stretching and toning.

For exercises performed while seated:

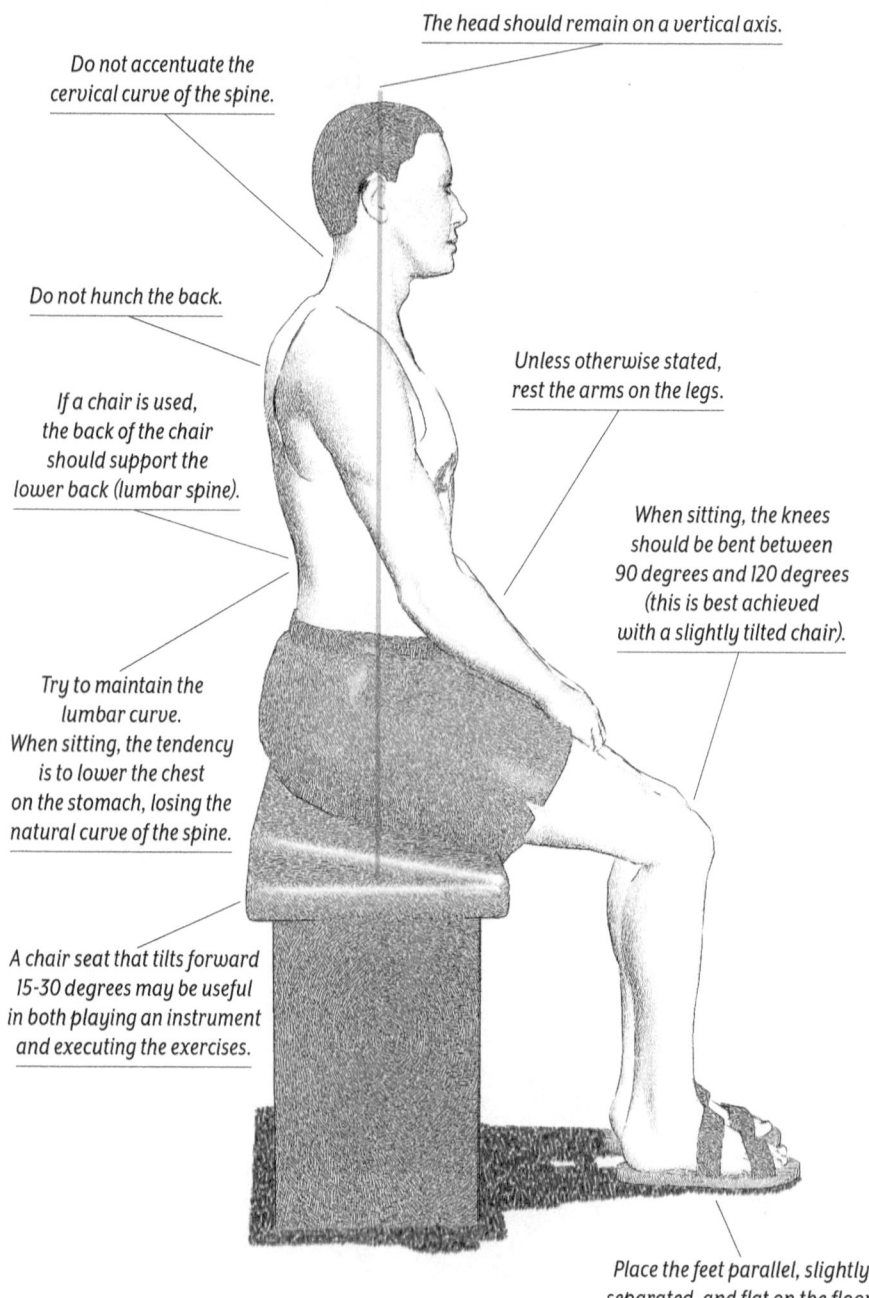

The head should remain on a vertical axis.

Do not accentuate the cervical curve of the spine.

Do not hunch the back.

If a chair is used, the back of the chair should support the lower back (lumbar spine).

Unless otherwise stated, rest the arms on the legs.

When sitting, the knees should be bent between 90 degrees and 120 degrees (this is best achieved with a slightly tilted chair).

Try to maintain the lumbar curve. When sitting, the tendency is to lower the chest on the stomach, losing the natural curve of the spine.

A chair seat that tilts forward 15-30 degrees may be useful in both playing an instrument and executing the exercises.

Place the feet parallel, slightly separated, and flat on the floor.

# CHAPTER TWO

**BASIC CONCEPTS**

*For exercises that are performed standing:*

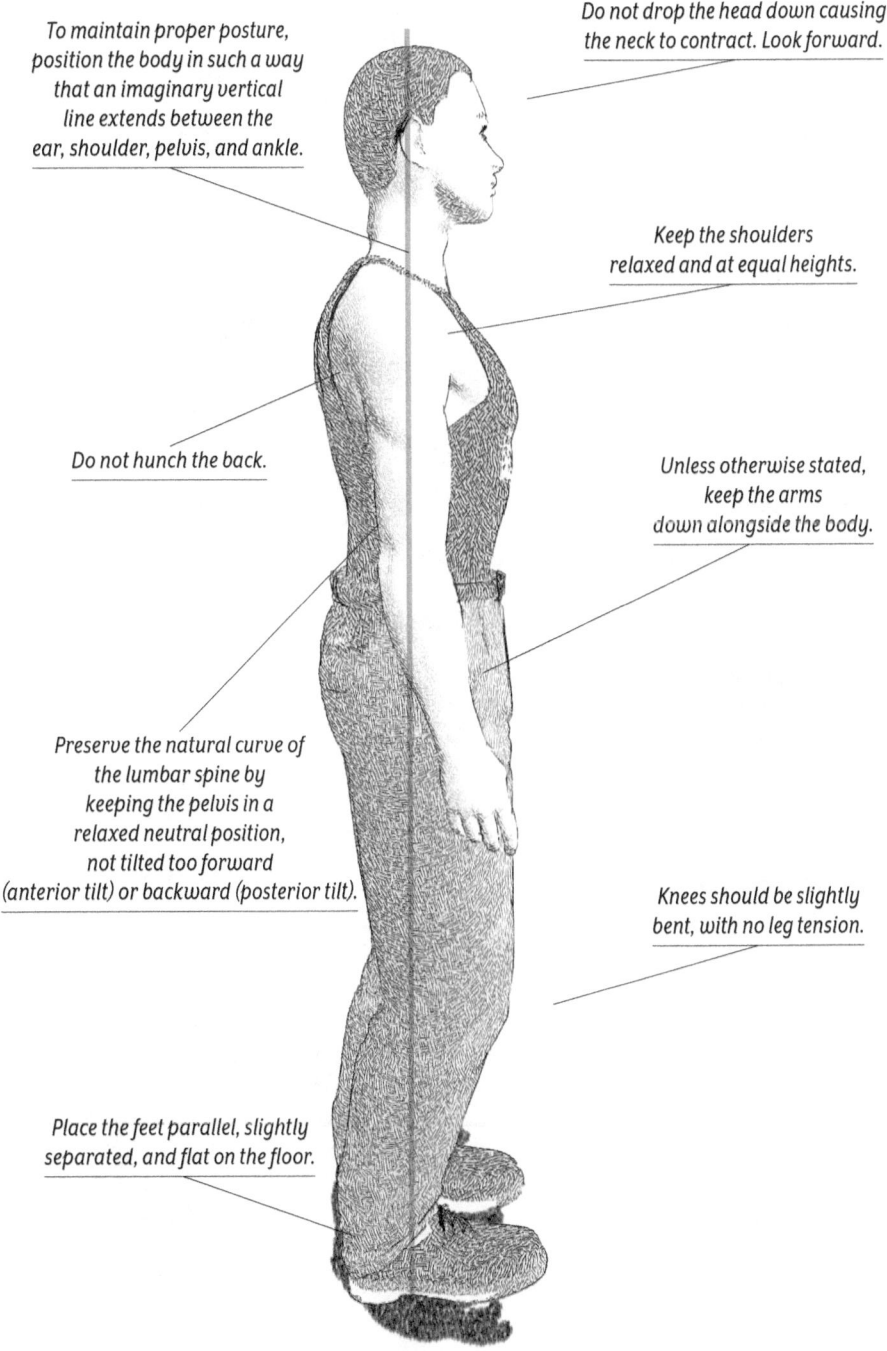

To maintain proper posture, position the body in such a way that an imaginary vertical line extends between the ear, shoulder, pelvis, and ankle.

Do not drop the head down causing the neck to contract. Look forward.

Keep the shoulders relaxed and at equal heights.

Do not hunch the back.

Unless otherwise stated, keep the arms down alongside the body.

Preserve the natural curve of the lumbar spine by keeping the pelvis in a relaxed neutral position, not tilted too forward (anterior tilt) or backward (posterior tilt).

Knees should be slightly bent, with no leg tension.

Place the feet parallel, slightly separated, and flat on the floor.

**Summary:**

Flexibility exercises for the musician:

- ▶ Improve muscle tone and elasticity as well as joint mobility and coordination.
- ▶ Prepare the muscles for stretching and playing, helping to maintain ample flexibility.
- ▶ Are a healthy way to gradually transition between rest and activity.
- ▶ Help to prevent injury.
- ▶ Should always be done before playing.
- ▶ Can be done anytime stiffness in the body is noticed.
- ▶ Do not require any special equipment or clothing.
- ▶ Require slow and rhythmic breathing.
- ▶ Necessitate smooth and gentle back and forth movements, avoiding pain.
- ▶ Should be a personal journey. Do not compare yourself with other musicians.
- ▶ Can be done anywhere.
- ▶ Can be done anytime.

CHAPTER TWO  BASIC CONCEPTS

# STRETCHING EXERCISES

**Definition:**

There are many different ways to stretch, each one having its own technique and effects. Stretches are maneuvers, performed either by yourself or assisted by a second person, designed to lengthen the tendons and muscles and act in a preventive or therapeutic manner.

Recently, some studies have doubted the positive, preventive effects of stretching and have pointed out that, in some cases, stretching can harm aspects of performance. It is not within the scope of this book to discuss this issue, but since it has generated confusion, mentioning a few key points may be appropriate.

New research shows that any negative effects of stretching are related only to maximum muscular effort or explosive movements in athletes. More research is necessary to confirm and better explain this data. In any case, these extreme actions are not used when playing a musical instrument. So musicians should not be concerned that the stretches proposed in this book will have any negative consequences on their muscular performance.

That being said, the most important advice for any exercise, whether included in this book or not, is that after trying it for a few days, assess which ways and to what degrees the exercise is beneficial. Based on this assessment, decide if the exercise should be adopted, adapted, or avoided.

The stretching exercises proposed in this book aim to lengthen the muscles and tendons by performing the opposite movement from that in which the muscle usually engages when activated.

Take, for example, a guitarist who has been working diligently on a piece containing many bar chord changes. In this case, the muscle that creates the *thumb flexion* of the left hand contributes to pressure on the neck of the guitar. It is necessary to offset the strain on the thumb through stretching. It would be useful for the guitarist to perform a stretch by *extending this finger* (6-Thumb back, page 33).

**Purpose:**

Generally, stretching can improve fitness and, by its relaxing effect, also the mental state of the musician. In particular, it contributes to a better understanding of the body allowing for enhanced performance and reduced muscle tension. Stretching also facilitates the body's understanding of motor activity, making work more rewarding and keeping the body agile and elastic.

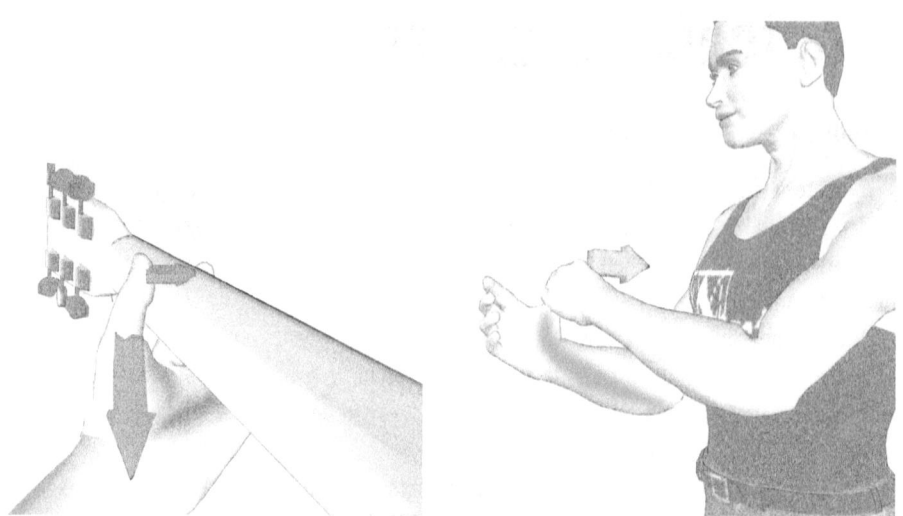

*The load on the flexor muscle of the thumb[31], due to playing pieces with many bar chords, can be adequately rebalanced through stretching in the opposite direction.*

Stretching helps keep muscles flexible and prepares them so that movements can be performed without excessive strain. Therefore, stretching before and after an activity maintains flexibility and helps prevent the most common injuries.

Stretching can improve performance and promote muscle restoration after playing via multiple mechanisms. However, only prominent ones are mentioned. Stretching before playing lengthens the muscles, leading to increased power and stamina. Heat is also created in the muscles and tendons, which increases flexibility and elasticity as well as lubricates the joints, giving freer mobility.

On the other hand, stretching reduces muscle tension, creating a sense of relaxation often beneficial to the musicians. When a muscle is stretched, the sensors between the muscle fibers are also stretched. This increases sensor perception leading to better coordination of movement. Thus, motor skills become more agile, free, and refined. This facilitates a more fruitful study, improved learning, and more optimal performance. Also, since stretching requires musicians to focus on the area they generally use to play their instrument, the development of body awareness is facilitated.

Stretching in the recovery phase helps eliminate stress that has accumulated in different parts of the body from playing. It aids the venous and lymphatic flow, helping to remove lactic acid build-up. This reduces muscle swelling and inflammation (one of the origins of muscle pain) and promotes recovery.

CHAPTER TWO                                                                          BASIC CONCEPTS

## Who Can Do This?

Stretching can be performed by anyone, or rather, should be performed by everyone (students, professionals, amateurs, teachers, etc.) whether they play a little or a great deal, and whether they have been injured or have always been healthy.

One limitation should be considered: it would be better for children who are flexible and who have not finished growing to avoid forcing the stretches and instead carry out the stretches in a very gentle way.

Following the basic rule that stretching should not cause pain ensures that these exercises have a low potential to cause harm. However, if you have an injury, seek medical advice (preferably from a professional who has experience working with musicians) to see if any of the exercises could be harmful.

## When and Where?

At a minimum, stretching should be performed before and after playing an instrument (including both practice and performance). It is best to make stretching a part of your daily practice routine. At first, it may be thought of as a burden that limits practice time. However, stretching will eventually be considered an essential part of practice just like tuning before playing or swabbing out moisture after playing.

Although it is advisable to stretch after briefly warming up the muscles (e.g., playing 5-10 minutes slowly and softly or doing flexibility exercises), no real restrictions apply.

It is obviously better to have a comfortable space and a relaxed atmosphere. Nevertheless, these exercises can be performed any time you want to reduce tension and facilitate the restoration of tissue.

The only situation in which it is not advised to stretch is right after eating. Although this advice is usually applied to exercises involving a much higher activity level, it is believed that digestion may be put under duress by the redistribution of blood that occurs when stretching. It should also be noted that exercises involving positions that can generate a small degree of tension in the abdomen (e.g., *23-Latissimus dorsi*, page 49, *43-Back*, page 66, *44-Lateral abdominal muscles*, page 67, *46-Spinal twist*, page 68, etc.) should be avoided right after eating as well.

Although in certain situations it will be necessary to adapt or shorten them, stretching exercises can be done anywhere even when time is limited; for example, during the intermission of a concert. Also, many situations outside the world of music offer great opportunities to fit in quality stretches such as: watching TV, waiting at a red light, working at the computer, or reading a book.

## Equipment:

You do not need any special equipment or clothing; however, a relaxed atmosphere, pleasant temperature, and comfortable loose clothing facilitate implementation. You should not be cold, nor should clothing limit mobility. Therefore, avoid wearing belts, sashes, or the like.

While performing the exercises, watching yourself in a mirror is suggested. This ensures the exercises are done correctly.

For floor exercises it is better, although not essential, to have a towel, blanket, or mat for general comfort.

## How to:

Stretching should be done to lengthen the muscles sufficiently (the movement and form is explained and illustrated for each stretch), but one must not do more than what is necessary. It is important to not force your body into position. Flexibility will improve with time: be patient and do not rush the process.

Luckily, the muscle will inform you whether it is being stretched too little or too much. If done slowly, keeping the rest of the body relaxed and concentrating on the muscle being stretched, you will be able to recognize when you are overexerting.

You should note a feeling of tension when stretching, but this should never be excessive. Do not cause pain and never bounce. Bouncing activates an unconscious and unintentional reaction of the body called stretch reflex. Stretch reflex is an automated nervous stimulation activated for the protection of the muscle to prevent excessive stress or an overly hasty movement that might result in injury. It involves a contraction that tries to counteract the excessive stretch. When you bounce or cause pain and activate this reflex, the opposite of the desired result is achieved (rather than relaxing and stretching, the muscle shortens and contracts). In addition, there is a small risk of injury that will eventually make the muscle less elastic.

To perform the stretch properly, it is beneficial to be relaxed and focused on the area of the body you are about to work. Breathing should be slow, rhythmic, and controlled. During the stretch, you must seek only a mild feeling of tension, which, if you are sufficiently relaxed, should decrease while maintaining the position. If the tension does not decrease, ease off slightly. From here slowly increase the stretch until you feel strong, but pleasant, tension. Hold for 20 to 30 seconds before releasing. If desired, this can be repeated as often as needed. Remember that you should stretch both sides (for example, first stretch the right arm and then the left, followed by the desired number of repetitions).

# CHAPTER TWO — BASIC CONCEPTS

It is advisable to stretch the more tense or overburdened side first. Typically people devote more time and attention to the muscle that they stretch first.

The range of motion needed for a proper stretch is extremely variable. Not only does it vary from one person to another, but within the same musician from one day to the next and one side of the body to the other. You may even find variations within the same day, as the muscles in the morning tend to be more rigid. In any case, the limit of stretching remains the sensation of pain, which should always be avoided.

The duration should also be based on individual perception. If you are feeling comfortable in the stretch, feel free to extend the holding time beyond the 30 seconds that is usually advised.

The figures in this book do not show how far a stretch should go, which can vary, rather how it should be performed (aspects that should be followed to the letter). Failing to use the correct technique may result in the use of a different, undesired muscle group.

The general position of the body for these exercises is the same as illustrated in the flexibility exercises section (pages 10 and 11).

**Summary:**

Stretching exercises for the musician:

- ▶ Prepare the muscles to perform and better tolerate the stress of playing.
- ▶ Contribute to muscle recovery after exercise.
- ▶ Help to prevent injuries.
- ▶ Do not need any special equipment.
- ▶ Should be performed in a relaxed and comfortable manner.
- ▶ Require slow, rhythmic, and controlled breathing.
- ▶ Should be performed without bouncing or jerking.
- ▶ Are to be performed free from pain and require only a pleasant amount of tension.
- ▶ Should not be thought of as a competition. Do not compare your stretches with other musicians.
- ▶ Are better begun on the side with the most stiffness or soreness (it is common to unconsciously spend more time on the side with which you start).

- ▶ Should be performed both before and after playing your instrument.
- ▶ Require consistency. It is relatively easy to remember to do them when feeling discomfort or tightness of muscles, but one tends to forget to do them when feeling good.
- ▶ Can be done anywhere.
- ▶ Can be done anytime.
- ▶ Should be held for 20-30 seconds on each side before repeating, if necessary.

# TONING EXERCISES

**Definition:**

In the 1950s and 1960s, muscle strength was considered the foundation of fitness. Because of this, most training regimens were based on building muscle. Although some of these same ideas and beliefs remain, today we have a more comprehensive concept of physical fitness. Modern fitness regimens reflect the need for improving cardiorespiratory endurance, musculoskeletal conditioning (strength, endurance, and flexibility), and balancing the various components that comprise our entire physical condition. Although they can be worked separately, strength (ability of the muscle to generate tension), endurance (ability of the muscle to apply a force repeatedly or maintain a prolonged muscle contraction), and flexibility are related to each other.

Cardiorespiratory endurance improves through physical activities involving large muscle groups. Recommended activities for musicians are: walking, dancing, skating, and cycling, among others (see Chapter 5 *Staying Healthy and Fit*, page 227).

Muscle strength, endurance, and, most importantly for musicians, balance can be improved through muscle toning exercises.

Although the exercises included in this book are primarily designed to maintain muscle condition, they can also be used to improve overall performance. It is a question of adequately adjusting their intensity and frequency.

To improve a muscle's strength, you must subject that muscle to appropriate workloads. These workloads should not be excessive, as this would overload the muscle; nor insufficient, since they would not initiate the desired change. To be effective, the workloads must be applied regularly.

Keep in mind that training is based on progression. If you recognize that your muscles permit you to do the exercises more easily, increase the intensity, speed, or repetitions. Decrease these parameters if you are finding the exercises too hard.

*8-Intrinsic plus* (page 34) or *28-Back to the wall* (page 53) are examples of toning exercises.

**Purpose:**

As mentioned, the basic objective of muscle toning for musicians is to offset imbalances that occur in everyday life and, most importantly, during musical activities (practicing, performing, etc.), thus reducing the risk of injury.

Cultivating strength, endurance, and muscle balance improves efficiency of movement, resulting in maximum performance while using minimal effort. Additionally, it helps

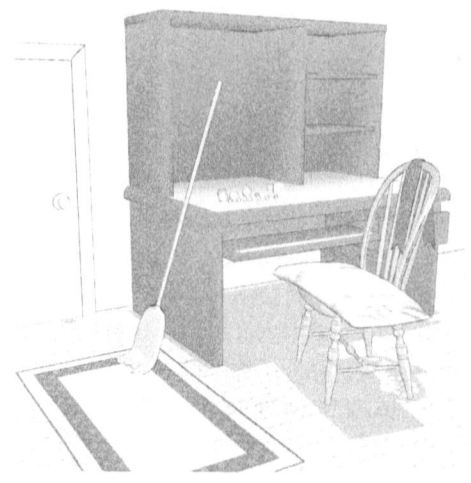

*The equipment necessary for toning exercises is affordable.*

to avoid bad posture, allowing you to better endure and adapt to heavier workloads while preserving and protecting the joints.

Musicians do not need to gain muscle volume or "bulk up" (known as muscle hypertrophy). This, aside from being unnecessary, could hinder your playing ability by making movements less fluid. The exercises proposed in this book are are aimed at simply toning, not muscle hypertrophy.

## Who Can Do This?

Although exercises that pose little risk to musicians have been carefully selected, toning exercises, unlike the stretching and flexibility exercises, are more demanding. These exercises are advised for all musicians, but it is important to avoid any that cause pain. If you have an injury or have had one in the past, seek medical advice (preferably from a professional who has experience working with musicians) to ensure these exercises will not aggravate it.

## When and Where?

Since toning exercises work the muscles, it is recommended to avoid them just before or after playing.

Our advice is to complete them a minimum of three times per week, if possible, leaving two hours of recovery time between exercising and playing your instrument.

In addition, if the aim is to improve overall physical performance, progressively increase the number of days, intensity, and number of repitições.

# CHAPTER TWO — BASIC CONCEPTS

Unlike the flexibility and stretching exercises, the toning exercises require a small amount of equipment, making it difficult to do these exercises just anywhere. However, you should not need a large financial investment in exercise machines or a gym membership. The equipment for toning exercises is affordable.

## Equipment:

You do not need a specific space or special clothing; however, a relaxed atmosphere, pleasant temperature, and comfortable loose clothing will make the process easier.

For floor exercises it is better, although not essential, to have a towel, blanket, or mat for general comfort.

You will need:

- 1 chair or stool.
- A wall or stable furniture for support.
- 8 small glass marbles (four per hand).
- 4 ping-pong balls (two per hand).
- 6 thin rubber bands about 1.25 inches (3 cm) in length (three per hand) – as strength improves, you can increase the thickness of the bands or use more of them to increase the resistance.
- 2 thicker rubber bands, about 2 inches (5 cm) in length (one per hand) – as strength improves, you can increase the thickness of the bands or use more of them to increase the resistance.
- 1 bed pillow.
- 1 stick (a broomstick works).
- 1 wide elastic band about 24 inches (60 cm) in length (usually purchased at sports stores and available in different resistances. The resistance level should be chosen based on your current degree of physical fitness).

## How to:

The proposed programs contain two types of toning exercises: isometric (performed by muscle contraction without movement, e.g., *26-Chair*, page 51) and isotonic (performed by muscle contraction with movement, e.g., *9-Rubber bands*, page 35).

Although each of the exercises described has specific guidelines, the following are basic concepts.

Isometric exercises generate a great deal of muscle fatigue. Therefore, the contraction should be short (about 6-10 seconds) with breaks of the same duration. The timing, frequency, and number of repetitions are indicated for each exercise (all having a minimum of 10 repetitions). This is not a maximum repetition exercise. Set a limit for yourself so as not to over-fatigue the muscles.

Isotonic exercises should be performed with smooth and slow movements. In order to prevent injury, be aware at all times of what you are doing and how you are performing the exercise. Also it is imperative to have a full and complete range of motion while maintaining constant muscle tension during the entirety of these exercises. For example, in exercise *27-Pole back* (page 52), use muscle tension not only when you raise the pole, but maintain that same tension while slowly returning the pole to the starting position (spend at least two seconds for the raising movement and two additional seconds for the returning movement). Doing the exercises this way gives you a more complete workout as well as helping to avoid possible injury.

If you find that you feel strong enough to complete more repetitions than the suggested amount, it is recommended that you take a short break before gradually adding the additional repetitions. Remember, musicians in general do not need large, overly developed muscles as this can limit flexibility and inhibit quick movements. Keep this in mind if you decide to go beyond the suggested repetitions.

Proper form and posture when performing these exercises are the same as illustrated in the flexibility exercises section (pages 10 and 11).

**Summary:**

Toning exercises for the musician:

- ▶ Preserve muscle fitness (both strength and endurance).
- ▶ Maintain balanced musculature.
- ▶ Improve musical performance.
- ▶ Prevent injury.
- ▶ Help to improve posture.
- ▶ Do not add muscle bulk.
- ▶ Should be performed by all musicians.

- ▶ Should not be done just before or after playing your instrument (2 to 3 hours of rest between playing and exercising).
- ▶ Should be performed a minimum of three days per week.
- ▶ Require little equipment.
- ▶ Are made up of isometric (muscles contract but no movement occurs) and isotonic exercises (muscles contract and movement occurs).
- ▶ As a general rule, isometric exercises should be held for about 6-10 seconds with a rest of about the same duration.
- ▶ As a general rule, isotonic exercises should be smooth and slow for both directions of the movement.

# WARMING UP AND COOLING DOWN

Instrumental performance involves the contraction and relaxation of dozens of muscles at high speeds over a period of time. This requires a constant energy intake and, consequently, output of metabolic waste. Blood circulation removes the metabolic waste. The more activity in which a given area of the body participates, the greater flow of blood it needs.

The total volume of blood in the body is constant. If you allocate a greater amount of blood to a particular area, that same amount must be subtracted from another area. The redistribution of blood does not happen instantaneously. If you start exercising a particular muscle or muscle group suddenly, your body will not be able to supply sufficient energy or oxygen to it immediately, resulting in a metabolic state known technically as anaerobic (without oxygen).

A muscle using an anaerobic metabolic pathway can withstand only a brief burst of explosive action, after which it becomes fatigued and prone to injury much more easily. More sustained activity requires establishing a pathway to an aerobic (with oxygen) metabolic state, which takes time to become fully operational. Without a gradual progression of activity allowing the establishment of proper blood circulation and aerobic metabolic activation, the muscle relies on the anaerobic metabolic pathways, resulting in lower energy and higher buildup of metabolic waste.

Executing a proper warm-up allows time for the aerobic metabolic pathways to open at full capacity and the blood supply to circulate adequately.

When muscle tissues are warm, metabolic reactions occur faster, nerve conduction is more agile, the muscle tissues themselves are more elastic, and joints are more fluid. This leads to faster and stronger muscle contraction. In addition, warming up is also a good way to psychologically prepare to play. For this reason, musicians should consider a proper warm-up to be an essential routine before playing.

## Warming up

Warming up has two phases: a general phase, unrelated to the specific musical activity that will be performed, in which the warm-up exercises use large muscle groups, and a specific phase with movements characteristic of the upcoming musical activity.

A general warm-up can be achieved through flexibility and stretching exercises. The specific warm-up should be based on a smooth and gradual progression on the instrument.

This means playing pieces of low difficulty that do not require extreme posture, positions, or force and are as varied as possible. The more difficult and intense the piece you need to play, the longer and more deliberate the warm-up should be.

For pianists, it may be appropriate to start with scales, so long as they are not performed across the entire keyboard or at high speeds. The correct way would be to play the scales at low speeds, and better yet, intersperse them with arpeggios. In fact, the more variety in the warm-up, the better.

String players should use a more relaxed and wide vibrato or work slowly on intonation without vibrato. The extreme high register, which puts their wrists in forced positions, should be avoided initially. The warm-up should not include strenuous techniques such as double stops or sautillé.

If, for whatever reason, you do not have an opportunity to do your warm-up routine (for example arriving just before a concert), you must try to warm up in some other way. One possibility is to move your fingers as if they were playing but not creating sound. Another option is to play a little more relaxed for the first few minutes (for instance, use a more relaxed vibrato with minimal pressure on the strings).

It would be ideal if specifically designated warm-up rooms were available for music students before class. Since this seems unlikely, it is at least advisable that the teacher devote the first few minutes to warming up. Both stretching and flexibility exercises work well in a group setting. The teacher could also begin class with a soft, easy piece that would serve as an adequate progression towards the more difficult pieces to be played later in class.

Similarly, orchestras should plan time for stretching and flexibility exercises before diving into progressively more difficult music.

**Cooling down**

It is not wise to suddenly stop playing once the day's work is finished. Cooling down allows the body in general, as well as the particular muscles that were worked, to more effectively remove metabolic waste and accumulated tension. This shortens the body's recovery time as well as prevents injuries caused by fatigue or metabolic waste accumulation.

Similar to warming up, cooling down also has two phases. The first is to gradually reduce the intensity, difficulty, and speed of the pieces played. If the activity of the day has been short or not intense, 5 minutes will suffice as a proper cool-down. Longer, more intense activity may require 10 to 20 minutes to properly cool down. The second phase should consist of specific stretches of the areas that were worked throughout the day.

In Chapter 4 *Exercises by Instrument* (page 87), exercises are proposed for a warm-up (identified as "before playing") and a cool-down (denoted as "after playing"). This chapter includes exercises that have been chosen according to the specific requirements of each instrument.

**Summary:**

Warming up:

- ▶ Increases muscular blood flow, nerve conduction velocity, joint mobility, and tissue elasticity.
- ▶ Leads to increased physical performance, less possibility of fatigue or injury, and a better psychological preparation for the activity.
- ▶ Has two phases: a general phase (flexibility and stretching exercises) and a specific phase (work on the instrument).
- ▶ Has important key points, including minimal pressure, variety, moderate speed, and neutral joint position.

Cooling down:

- ▶ Allows for a faster recovery times, helps to eliminate metabolic waste, and prevents injury or fatigue.
- ▶ Consists of two phases: a general phase (gradual decline in activity) and a specific phase (stretching of specifically worked areas).

Chapter Three

# EXERCISES BY REGION OF THE BODY

**IN TUNE**

Because of the demands of musical activity on each of the body's zones, exercises are presented here that counterbalance the stresses these areas withstand. Also included are flexibility and stretching exercises for preparing an area before an activity or for restoring it to equilibrium afterwards, as well as strengthening exercises for reconditioning zones that are often weakened or imbalanced in musicians.

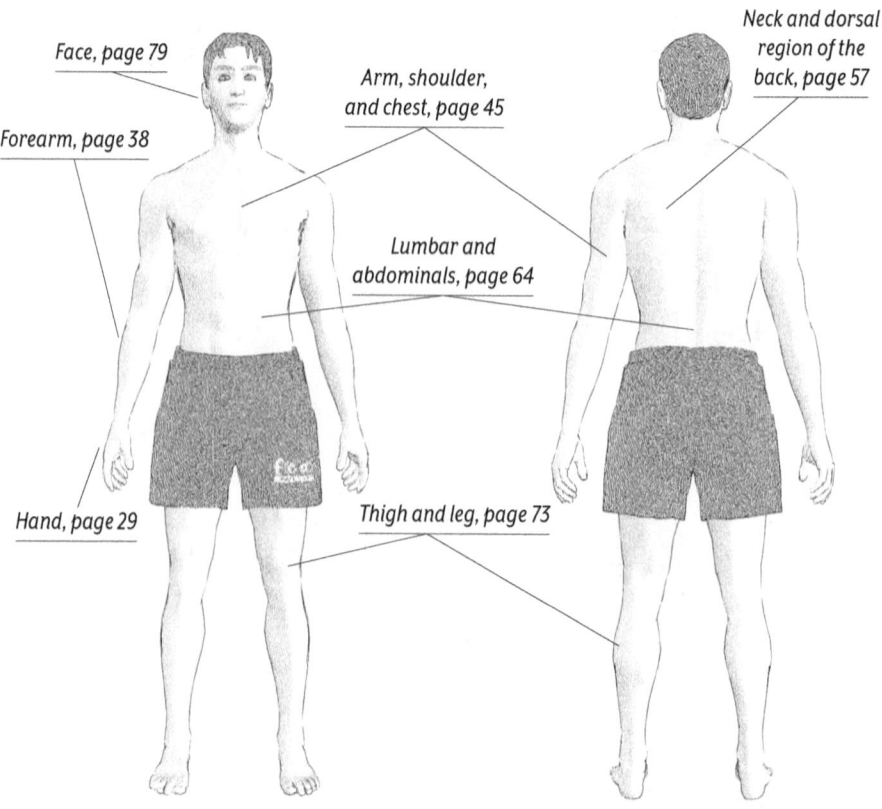

*Face, page 79*

*Forearm, page 38*

*Arm, shoulder, and chest, page 45*

*Neck and dorsal region of the back, page 57*

*Lumbar and abdominals, page 64*

*Hand, page 29*

*Thigh and leg, page 73*

# CHAPTER THREE

EXERCISES BY REGION OF THE BODY

# HAND

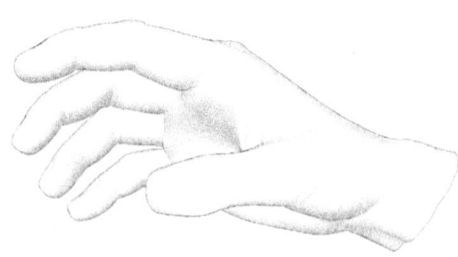

It is obvious that a musician's work on an instrument gives the hands exceptional dexterity and agility. The problem is that some muscles become more developed to the detriment of others. This is the case of the extensor and flexor muscles of the fingers and the extensor and flexor muscles of the wrist (mainly the *flexor carpi ulnaris*[8], the *extensor digitorum communis*[7] and *flexor digitorum profundus*[9], and the *radial muscles*[25], versus the intrinsic muscles of the hand (*dorsal interossei*[6], *palmar interossei*[19]) and the *lumbricals of the hand*[15].

Taking care of these intrinsic muscles by doing flexibility and stretching exercises prior to playing, stretching exercises after playing, and strengthening and toning exercises to gain strength in the area makes it possible for a musician to work in a more balanced and healthy manner.

In addition, these exercises will provide a wider range of movement, better coordination and independence of the fingers.

## FLEXIBILITY EXERCISES

**1   Finger mobility 1**

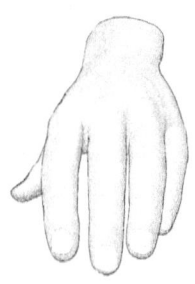

Finger movement is achieved by means of two muscle groups: those in the forearm (which control the fingers by means of tendons) and those in the hand (intrinsic hand muscles). This exercise specifically prepares the intrinsic hand muscles for work.

**Initial position:** Seated or standing with your arms relaxed in front of you. Rest your hands on your thighs if standing, or on a table if seated.

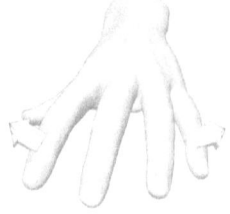

**Workout:** Slowly separate the fingers from each other as much as possible (abduction), and then bring them together (adduction). Repeat 10 to 15 times. You can also try to separate them one by one.

**Attention:** The hand must be kept totally relaxed in order not to strain the muscles during the exercise.

## 2 Finger mobility 2

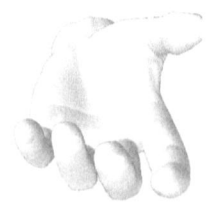

This exercise works the muscles in the hand (intrinsic hand muscles) as well as those in the forearm.

**Initial position:** Seated or standing with your arms relaxed in front of you. Rest your hands on your thighs if standing, or on a table if seated.

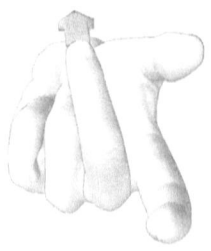

**Workout:** *Flex your fingers* one by one until your hand is closed (do not move all of your fingers at the same time, but rather when one is being flexed the others must be kept still). Once all fingers have been flexed (making a fist), *extend* them one by one. Repeat 10 to 15 times.

**Attention:** Do not strain when doing this exercise; these are merely movement exercises. The tendon connections between fingers make it anatomically impossible to move one finger and keep the others completely still. Do not worry if the non-flexing fingers do not remain completely still and and do not forcefully prevent these movements.

| CHAPTER THREE | EXERCISES BY REGION OF THE BODY |

## STRETCHING EXERCISES

### 3   Hand muscles

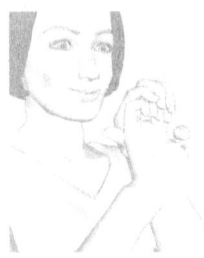

The intrinsic muscles (such as the *dorsal interossei*[6], *palmar interossei*[19] and the *lumbricals of the hand*[15]) are located between the bones of the hand and are crucial for finger mobility. It is necessary to counterbalance the stresses they withstand when playing an instrument.

**Initial position:** Lift your stretched fingers and wrist slightly backward (similar to indicating to someone to stop). The palm of your hand must be facing forward. Using your opposite hand, grasp the finger you want to stretch by placing the *proximal interphalangeal joint* and the *distal interphalangeal joint* in *flexion*.

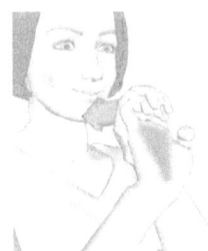

**Stretch:** Keeping your *fingers in flexion*, pull one finger back at a time (*extension* of the *metacarpophalangeal joint*). Hold the stretch for 20 seconds. Do this for each finger on both hands except for the thumb.

**Attention:** This stretch may cause slight pain at the base of the fingers in hands that are not flexible. If this is the case, it is better not to do it. However, once you can control the stretch being done in each finger, you can do this exercise by taking back all of the fingers at the same time as shown in the figure.

### 4   Palm of the hand

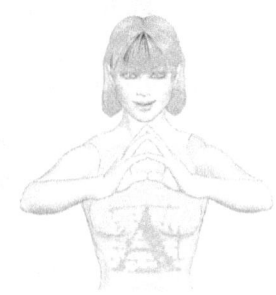

The palmar aponeurosis is a fibrous structure that takes up almost the entire palm of the hand and aids in *finger flexion*. As this part of the hand is usually contracted when playing an instrument, it is recommended to stretch it regularly.

**Initial position:** Join the fingertips of both hands while keeping the heels of both hands separate and your elbows up.

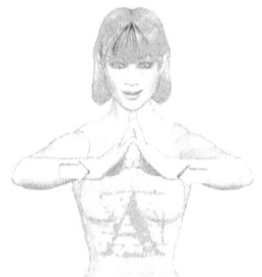

**Stretch:** Press one hand against the other trying to bring the base of the fingers together (making a maximum *extension* of the *metacarpophalangeal joint*) without changing the position of the wrist and elbows. Hold the stretch for 20 seconds.

**Attention:** Do not overly strain when doing this exercise since this can easily cause pain. Do not join the heels of the hands together or raise your elbows excessively.

## 5    Thumb down

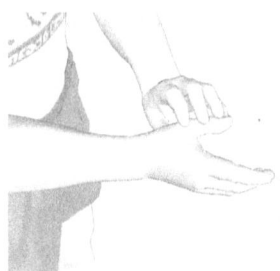

The muscles that *extend the thumb* (including the *short extensor of the thumb*[18]) help stabilize the thumb and especially suffer when the wrist is working in strained positions. Since these hazardous situations are common when playing an instrument, stretching helps maintain health.

**Initial position:** Stretch your arm out in front of you (*elbow extension*) at approximately waist height with your palm facing inwards (thumb on top). Grasp your thumb with the fingertips of your opposite hand so that your four fingers are above and the thumb is below.

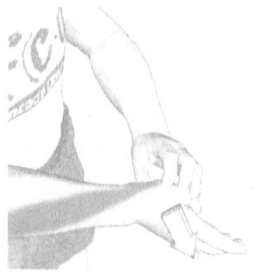

**Stretch:** Press your thumb down (*flexion*) also bending your wrist in the same direction (*ulnar deviation*). Hold the stretch for 20 seconds. Do the same movement with the opposite hand. You can try doing the stretch by adding an *internal arm* and *hand rotation*.

**Attention**: It is necessary to bend the entire thumb starting from the tip.

## CHAPTER THREE — EXERCISES BY REGION OF THE BODY

## 6   Thumb back

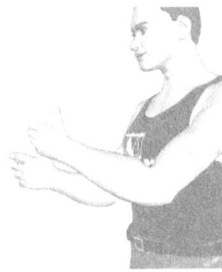

The muscles that let you *flex the thumb*, the small muscles at the base (primarily the *short flexor of the thumb*[31]) as well as the larger muscles in the forearm, are generally worked intensely in musicians. This exercise stretches all of these muscles.

**Initial position:** Either standing or seated with your *elbow flexed* (bent) and your thumb pointing up, take your thumb with the palm of the opposite hand.

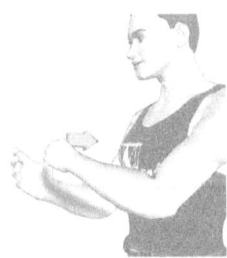

**Stretch:** Pull your thumb back. It is preferable for it to be towards your body rather than in the direction of your arm. Hold the stretch for 20 seconds in each hand.

---

**Attention:** It is necessary to stretch the entire finger [thumb], including the tip, and keep the wrist from moving. Musicians who have excessive mobility of the *metacarpophalangeal joint* of their thumb, as shown in the figure below, should try not to strain their thumb.

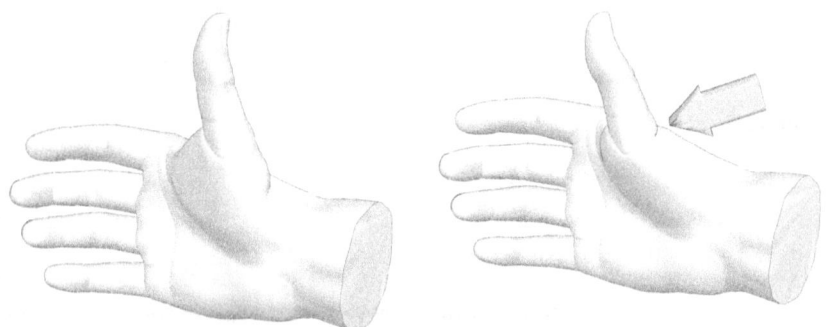

*Many musicians have an exceedingly high mobility of the joint at the base of the thumb (metacarpophalangeal). When they extend their thumb instead of moving as a unit (figure on the left), the thumb extends from this joint. When doing this exercise, these musicians should try to avoid accentuating the excessive mobility of the joint.*

## TONING EXERCISES

### 7   Picking up marbles

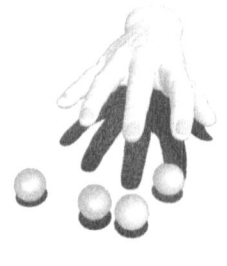

Marble exercises for the hand (*dorsal interossei*[6], *palmar interossei*[19], and the *lumbricals of the hand*[15]) combine toning and coordination, both of which are useful for musicians.

**Initial position:** Seated in front of a table or a smooth surface, place four glass marbles on the table.

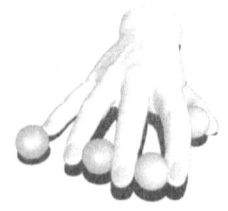

**Workout:** With your hand open, pick up the marbles one by one between the tips of your fingers, near the fingernails. Once all of the marbles have been picked up, squeeze them between your fingers without straining. Hold for 5-6 seconds and then let them go, again one by one. Do this exercise for 3 minutes per hand. If your hands are sufficiently agile, you can do both hands at the same time.

**Attention:** It is advisable to alternate the finger with which you start. Begin the exercise one time with the little finger and the next time with the thumb or any other finger. When releasing the marbles, you should also alternate the side from which you begin. It is important to keep your fingers straight to prevent *hyperextension*, especially for musicians who have increased joint mobility (*hypermobility*). You can also use different sized marbles and hold them at varying points of the fingers.

### 8   Intrinsic plus

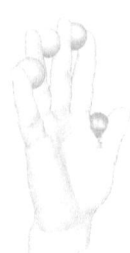

This exercise is a good way to tone hand muscles and to make up for the imbalance that generally occurs when playing a musical instrument.

**Initial position:** Seated in front of a table or a smooth surface, place four glass marbles on the table. Pick up one between each finger close to the tips of the fingers then raise the hand up.

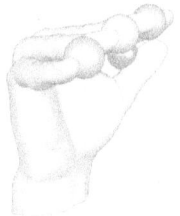

**Workout:** While keeping the fingers fully stretched, slowly *flex* the *metacarpophalangeal joint* as far as you can. Then return to the initial position. Do this exercise for 3 minutes per hand. If your hands are sufficiently agile, the exercise can be done with both hands at the same time.

**Attention:** Do not *flex the wrist* since this would be working the muscles in the forearm and not the hand muscles (the intrinsic muscles). Always keep your fingers straight. You can also use different sized marbles and hold them at varying points of the fingers.

## 9  Rubber bands

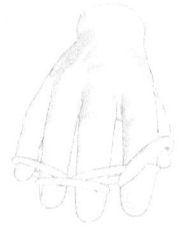

Working the intrinsic hand muscles (*dorsal interossei*[6], *palmar interossei*[19], and the *lumbricals of the hand*[15]) against resistance keeps them better prepared to withstand the stresses of playing and prevents injuries.

**Initial position:** Seated in front of a table or a smooth surface, place a large rubber band between your thumb and the index finger and smaller bands on each pair of your other fingers (index finger – middle finger, middle finger – ring finger, and ring finger – little finger). Keep your hand supported on the table.

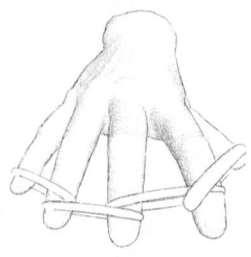

**Workout:** Spread your fingers slightly, tensing the rubber bands, and hold the position for 5 or 6 seconds. Then return to the intitial position. Do this exercise for 3 minutes per hand. If your hands are sufficiently agile, the exercise can be done with both hands at the same time.

**Attention:** When spreading your fingers, it is important not to raise your fingertips off the surface. That would work the muscles of the forearm rather than the hand muscles, which are the ones of interest here. You do not need to excessively spread your fingers, just create a slight tension in the rubber bands. You can also use different rubber bands (tighter or looser) and place them at varying points of your fingers.

## 10  Ball juggling

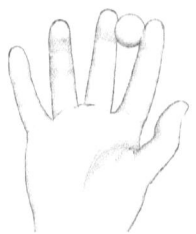

This agility exercise puts your fingers through their paces. It is a great toning and coordination exercise for musicians and will demonstrate that your skill on an instrument does not automatically give you an edge in all exercises.

**Initial position:** Seated or standing. You will need a rubber ball measuring at most 1.25 inches (3 cm) in diameter. Place the ball between two of your fingers.

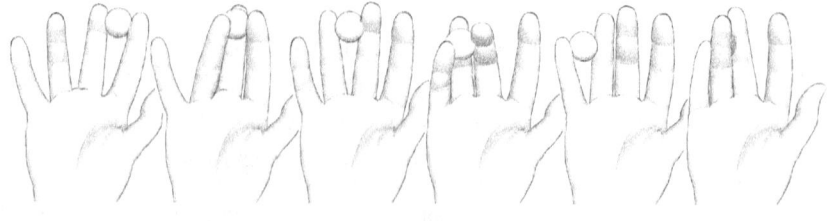

**Workout:** The finger located next to the ones holding the ball moves over to get the ball. After the ball has been passed from finger to finger, repeat until the ball has traveled to all fingers. Then pass the ball back along the backside of your fingers. The ball should first travel in front of the fingers and come back behind them. This exercise should be done for 3 minutes per hand. If your hands are sufficiently agile, the exercise can be done with both hands at the same time. You can also do a variation where you pass the ball in front of one finger and behind the next or create new and different patterns each time. The thumb may also be included when passing the ball back and forth.

**Attention:** Try to keep your hand relaxed and do not be discouraged if at the beginning you drop the ball frequently.

# CHAPTER THREE
## EXERCISES BY REGION OF THE BODY

## 11  Ping-pong balls

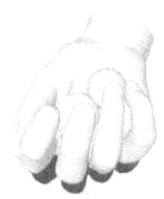

This exercise is a good way to combine relaxation with working out a number of the muscles involved in hand movements.

**Initial position:** Seated or standing. Place two ping-pong balls (or similarly sized balls) in the palm of your hand with your fingers slightly *flexed* over them.

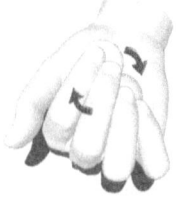

**Workout:** Try to get the ping-pong balls to rotate in your palm by means of *flexion/extension of the fingers*, first one direction and then the other. This exercise should be done for 3 minutes per hand. If your hands are sufficiently agile, the exercise can be done with both hands at the same time.

---

**Attention:** The balls must always be touching. One direction is usually easier than the other, but try to rotate them in both directions. In any case, if one way causes excessive stress, it is better to stop and only rotate them toward the easier side.

# FOREARM

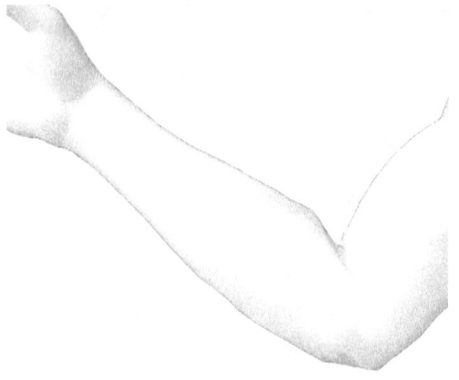

The forearm muscles are used in all movements and gestures made by musicians who perform with their upper extremities (use of the fingers, wrist, and elbow). This also involves a set of muscles that combine dynamic action (alternating movement of the fingers) with a type of isometrics (stabilization of the joints), making them more prone to overstress. It is not recommended (except in specific circumstances) to strengthen these muscles, since they are sufficiently developed by playing a musical instrument. However, it is crucial to counterbalance these stresses with a flexibility workout before playing, and stretches before and after playing.

## FLEXIBILITY EXERCISES

**12  Full arm rotations**

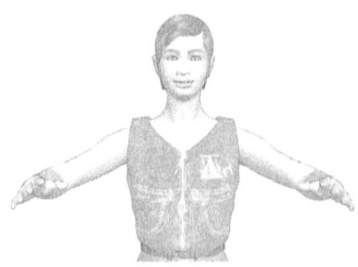

This exercise combines movements in all joints (fingers, wrists, elbows, and shoulders). This way the entire upper body is being prepared for work at the same time.

**Initial position:** Seated or standing, feet firmly planted on the ground with the spinal column as straight as possible and your arms out in front. Begin by *extending your fingers*, with your *wrists slightly extended* and your *elbows flexed* (bent) and away from your body.

| CHAPTER THREE | EXERCISES BY REGION OF THE BODY |

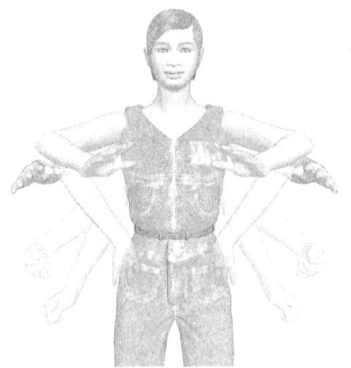

**Workout:** Rotate your arms in a forward motion. This exercise simulates the butterfly stroke, adding the opening and closing of your hands and *extending* and *flexing your wrist* in each cycle. Repeat 10 times, and then perform the exercise in the opposite direction. Begin the *flexion of the fingers* and *wrists* as your arms travel behind you.

**Attention:** If you have shoulder problems, only rotate from the elbow, continuing to utilize the wrist and finger movements. You can also modify the pattern by combining different movements. For instance, first bend the fingers while *flexing the wrists*, then *extend the fingers* while *flexing the wrist*.

## STRETCHING EXERCISES

### 13 Wrist down

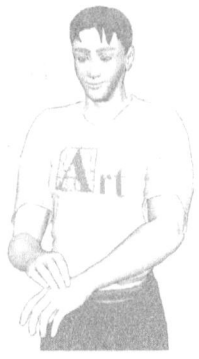

The *extensor digitorum communis*[7] and *radial muscles*[25] stabilize the wrist and *extend the fingers*. Musicians often work them in sustained and contracted positions (isometric). The result is that they easily become overstressed, so it is important to remember to stretch them.

**Initial position:** Put your arm out with your elbow slightly *flexed* (bent) with the palm of your hand facing down. Grab the back of your hand in between second and third fingers.

**IN TUNE**

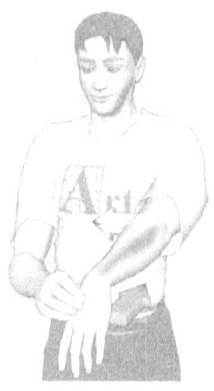

**Stretch:** *Flex your wrist* downwards by pushing on the back of your hand. Simultaneously, *extend your elbow* and hold the stretch for 20 seconds per hand. The stretch can be increased by adding an *internal rotation* (rotating the forearm in).

**Attention:** Keep the fingers of the hand that is being stretched totally relaxed. You can change the degree of flexion of your elbow on each repetition to better stretch the different parts of these muscles.

## 14  Fist out

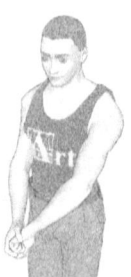

Of the muscles in the forearm, the *extensor digitorum communis*[7] has the greatest tendency to accumulate stress when playing. For this reason, it should be stretched regularly.

**Initial position:** Put out your arm with your *elbow slightly bent* and *internally rotated*, the palm of the hand facing out to the side. Make a fist with your thumb inside the other fingers. Enclose the fist with your opposite hand.

**Stretch:** *Flex your wrist* while *extending your elbow*. Hold the stretch for 20 seconds on each side.

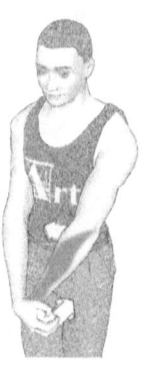

**Attention:** By varying the rotation of the forearm and the position of the elbow, the muscle zone that is being stretched changes. It is necessary to experiment to see which position results in a more thorough stretch. However, do not stretch only in that position. Always change, in some degree, the angle of the different joints that are involved. There should not be strain in any zone being stretched; only the muscle that is helping perform the stretch should be engaged.

## 15 Fist in

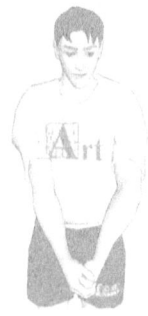

In musicians, the *extensor digitorum communis*[7] has a tendency to accumulate stress. Depending on the position of the forearm, it is possible to stretch one part more than another. This exercise is performed with *external rotation*.

**Initial position:** Put out your arm with your *elbow slightly bent* and the palm of your hand facing in. Make a fist with your thumb inside your other fingers. Grab the fist, covering the knuckles with your palm.

**Stretch:** With your opposite hand, try to increase the *flexion of the wrist* while *extending the elbow*. Hold the stretch for 20 seconds on each side.

**Attention:** Concentrate on how pressure is being applied to your hand and preferably try to concentrate the pressure on the 5th (little) finger area.

## 16 Hand back

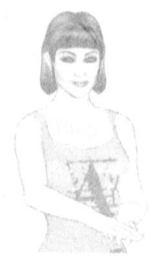

The flexor muscles of your fingers and wrist (mainly the *flexor digitorum profundus*[9] and the *flexor carpi ulnaris*[8]) accumulate stress due to repetitive motions, even though they generally alternate between contraction and relaxation. This results in the muscle fibers — as well as their tendons — being prone to overload if no preventative steps are taken.

**Initial position:** With your *elbow slightly bent* and your palm facing towards you, straighten your fingers (*extension*). Put the opposite hand perpendicular below the fingers with your palm facing up.

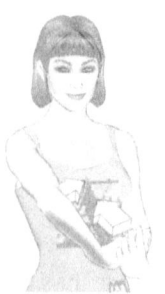

**Stretch:** *Straighten your elbow* while *extending your wrist* and *fingers* inwardly with your opposite hand. Hold the stretch for 20 seconds on each side.

**Attention:** Do not strain any area of your arm that is being stretched; just the muscle of the arm that is helping perform the stretch should be engaged. Do not do this stretch with your arms high and do not raise your shoulders. If you feel pain in the forearm that is helping perform the stretch, it is better to substitute a wall or some other solid object. In this case try not to exert pressure near your wrist.

## 17 Hand down

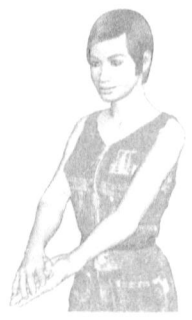

The flexor muscles of your fingers and wrist (mainly the *flexor digitorum profundus*[9] and the *flexor carpi ulnaris*[8]) can also be worked in an *external rotation*, which allows zones other than those of the previous exercise to be better stretched.

**Initial position:** With your *elbow slightly bent* and your palm facing up (*external rotation*), hold the fingers of your upturned hand with the opposite hand so that your palms are facing each other.

| CHAPTER THREE | EXERCISES BY REGION OF THE BODY |

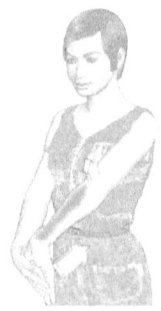

**Stretch:** Increase the *extension of your wrist* and *fingers* with your opposite hand. Hold the stretch for 20 seconds. Repeat on both sides. To make the stretch more intense, you can also *extend your elbow*. It is recommended to vary the degree of *elbow extension* for each repetition or during the exercise.

**Attention:** If you already noted a good deal of tension with *16 – Hand back*, it will not be necessary to do *17-Hand down*, since it is much more intense.

## 18  Hand inclined

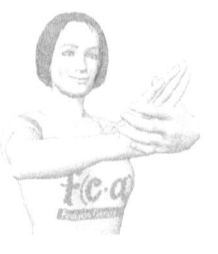

The *flexor carpi ulnaris*[8] is used by musicians in all wrist lateral movements and for stabilizing the wrist. Keeping it toned prevents problems and improves performance.

**Initial position:** Place the arm in *internal rotation*, the palm of the hand facing down and *elbows slightly bent*. Grab the palm of the hand.

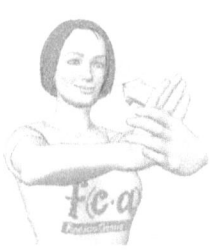

**Stretch:** It is necessary to combine two movements: the *extension of the wrist* and the *radial deviation* (tilt the hand laterally to the side towards your thumb). Hold the stretch for 20 seconds on each arm.

**Attention:** If sufficient pressure is not exerted on the thumb, only the flexor muscles of the fingers and of the wrist will be stretched but not the *flexor carpi ulnaris*[8].

**IN TUNE**

## TONING EXERCISES

Most of the muscle mass that moves the fingers in the hand is in the forearm. This is why some of the exercises done with the hand also help strengthen the muscles of the forearm. Previously mentioned hand exercises, *10-Ball juggling* and *11-Ping-pong balls*, will be sufficient for exercising this zone.

**CHAPTER THREE**  EXERCISES BY REGION OF THE BODY

# ARM, SHOULDER, AND CHEST

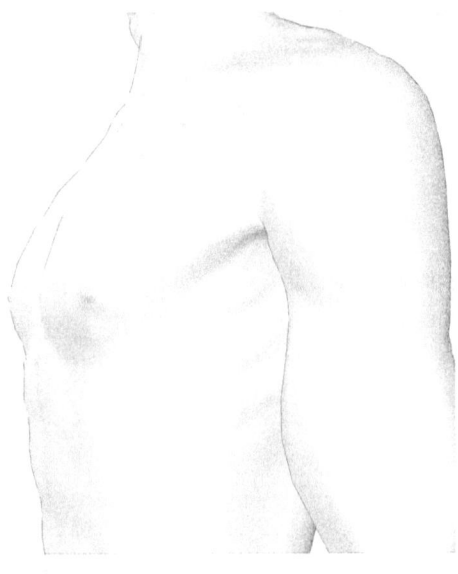

The arm muscles control both the position and the stabilization of the elbow and shoulder. They are essential for the hand to be able to act with the precision and freedom necessary to play.

Furthermore, the elbow often works in *flexion*. This tends to overstress the muscles, making it important to do flexibility exercises and stretches to counteract the stress.

Your shoulder is one of the joints in your body with the greatest mobility. However, this range of freedom comes at the cost of significant instability that must be counterbalanced with good muscle support.

The resulting problem of playing an instrument along with daily activity is that musicians generally use muscles that raise the shoulders to the detriment of those that lower them.

When determining how to avoid problems in this area, it is important to incorporate flexibility exercises before playing and stretches before and after playing, as well as a maintenance program that includes toning exercises for those muscles that draw the shoulders down.

## FLEXIBILITY EXERCISES

The exercise *12–Full arm rotation* incorporates not only movement of the wrist and forearm muscles but also of the elbow, shoulder, and other muscles in this zone. It is therefore a complete flexibility exercise for the entire upper body.

The following exercises are also recommended:

## 19 Raising and lowering the shoulders

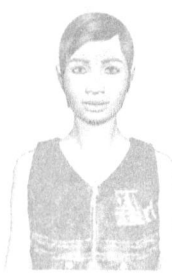

The shoulder area generally accumulates a great deal of stress when playing an instrument. This exercise is useful for preventing this stress since it warms up the structures involved and improves awareness.

**Initial position:** Sit or stand with your feet firmly planted on the ground. Your back must be as straight as possible and your arms should be relaxed and in front of you.

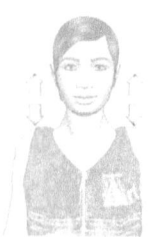

**Workout:** Raise your shoulders as far as you can, then slowly lower them so they are fully relaxed. The shoulders can be raised together, one at a time, or with a slight delay between the start of each side. Repeat this 10 or 15 times.

**Attention:** Do not strain the muscles in this area or cause tension. Make sure that your shoulders are totally relaxed at the end of the lowering phase.

## 20 Twisting the chest and arms

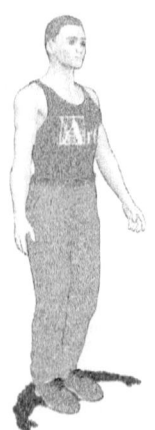

This exercise makes it possible to stretch the spinal column and the arms at the same time. In order to warm up and achieve good elasticity, it is crucial to perform this totally relaxed.

**Initial position:** Stand with your feet firmly planted on the ground and your back as straight as possible. Straighten your arms and hold them slightly away from your body.

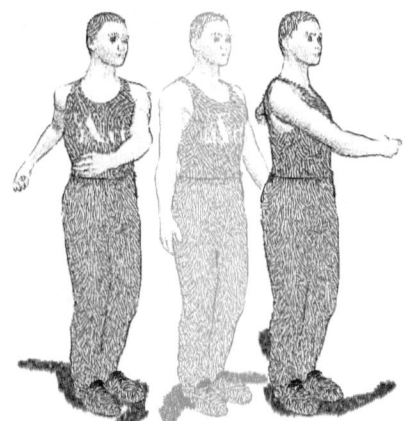

**Workout:** In a twisting motion, rotate your entire spinal column, first to one side and then slowly to the other. To make the rotation fluid, move your arms in the same direction as the twist. Repeat this 10 times.

**Attention:** The entire back should move independently from the pelvic area, which must remain stationary. To prevent dizziness, keep your eyes looking forward during the entire exercise.

## STRETCHING EXERCISES

### 21 Chest

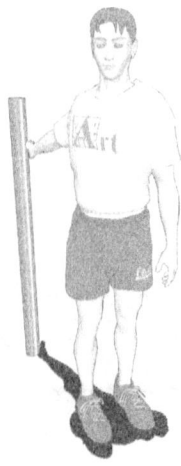

The anterior muscles of the arms and chest (primarily *biceps*[3] and *pectoral muscles*[21]) gradually accumulate stress from playing, especially when playing involves *closing the shoulders*. Stretching them helps you maintain a better posture and reduce tension.

**Initial position:** Stand next to a wall or sturdy object. Fully *extend* your arm back, supporting the palm of your hand on the wall or object. Keep your feet facing forward while your arm is behind you. The upper part of your chest will be twisted.

# IN TUNE

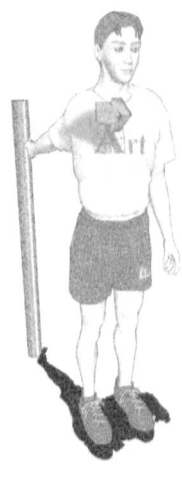

**Stretch:** For the side that you are stretching, pull the shoulder forward as if you are trying to return your chest to its natural forward-facing position. While keeping your hand pressed against the wall or object, hold the stretch for 20 seconds per side.

**Attention:** It is not advisable to exercise both arms at the same time since this generally entails a lower back position that is not recommended (page 254). Keep your hand open and high enough to feel tension in your arm and chest. Never raise it above shoulder height since this can cause an injury. Be careful with this exercise if you have ever dislocated your shoulder.

## 22 Posterior arm muscles

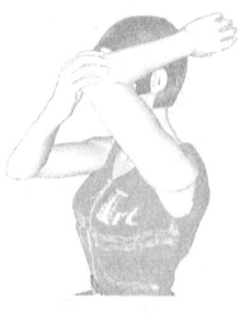

The muscles in the back of your arm (primarily the *triceps brachii*[35]) help stabilize the shoulder and elbow. As they are generally contracted when playing an instrument, it is good to stretch them to restore their length.

**Initial position:** Stand with your feet slightly apart. Place the arm you want to stretch with the *elbow slightly bent* at face height with your hand behind your shoulder. With your opposite hand, clasp your elbow.

**Stretch:** Pull your elbow back to increase its *flexion*. Hold the stretch for 20 seconds per side.

**Attention:** If you have problems with your shoulder tendons, it is better not to do this exercise since they could be pinched. Try to keep your lower back flat (avoid *hyperlordosis*); otherwise, this area can be overstressed. The degree at which you *bend your elbow* will determine the level of stretch. Keep this in mind. On the other hand, if you feel pain in your forearms, you can press your elbow against a wall instead of using your other arm.

## 23 Latissimus dorsi

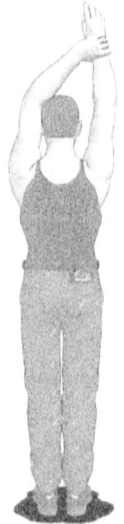

The *latissimus dorsi*[13] is the large muscle that starts at the back and goes to the arm at shoulder height. Stretching it helps restore mobility to the shoulder and maintains an equilibrium of muscle tone in the back.

**Initial position:** Stand with your feet slightly apart. Fully extend one arm above your head and slightly behind it. With your opposite hand, grab your arm near the wrist or elbow.

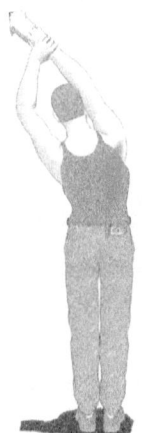

**Stretch:** Pull up on the stretched arm and slightly bend to the opposite side. Hold the stretch for 20 seconds per side.

# IN TUNE

**Attention:** You should feel tension in your arm and in your side, but not in your back. This exercise is not recommended if you have shoulder problems. Try not to arch the lower part of your back (avoid *hyperlordosis*).

## 24  Rear shoulder

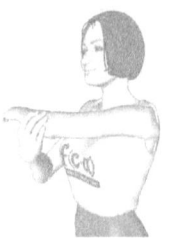

Many instruments require the musician to often use the *posterior deltoid*[22]. Therefore, this muscle should be stretched regularly.

**Initial position:** While standing, raise your arm in front of you at chest height with your *elbow bent* and palm facing down. Grasp your elbow from below with your opposite hand.

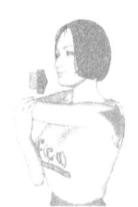

**Stretch:** Push your arm towards the opposite shoulder making sure that arm travels above that shoulder, as if you were trying to hug yourself. Hold the stretch for 20 seconds per arm.

**Attention:** Be careful with this exercise if you have problems with your shoulder tendons. Do not do this exercise if you feel any pain while performing it, especially pain in the front of the shoulder.

# TONING EXERCISES

## 25  Pillow

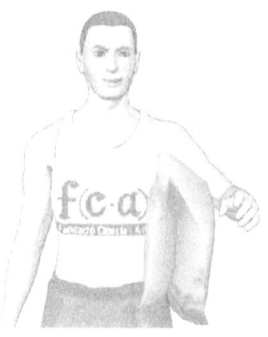

Most of the movements made when playing an instrument (as well as in daily life) involve raising at least one arm and keeping it raised. This results in shoulder imbalance which must be counterbalanced with shoulder drop exercises, like this one.

**Initial position:** Standing or seated in a chair with no armrests, with your feet firmly planted on the ground

**CHAPTER THREE**      **EXERCISES BY REGION OF THE BODY**

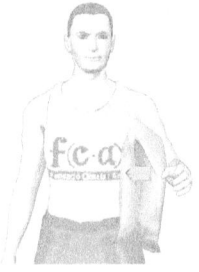

and your back straight. Place a pillow between your arm and chest, keeping your *elbow bent* 90°.

**Workout:** With your elbow, press the pillow against your body for 6 seconds followed by a 6-second rest. Repeat this for 5 minutes. This exercise can be done with both arms simultaneously. From repetition to repetition, the intensity with which you press the pillow to your body can be varied. Within any given repetition, the intensity may also vary from start to finish.

**Attention:** Do not press your hand against your abdomen since the forearm must, at all times, be perpendicular to your body, with your fingers pointing forward.

## 26 Chair

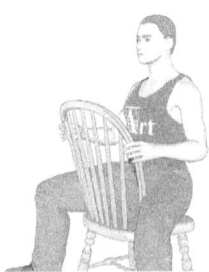

To counterbalance the asymmetrical activity of the shoulder muscles, it is desirable to strengthen the muscles that help lower your shoulders. In this case, a chair or similar object can be used.

**Initial position:** Seated backward in a chair (or with another chair with its back placed in front of you). Grab each side of the back of the chair with your hands.

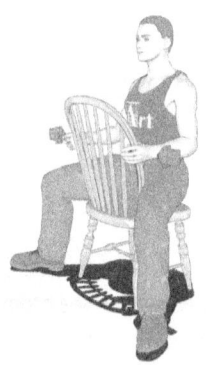

**Workout:** Push in against the chair as if you wanted to break it between your hands. You should keep your elbows close to your body. Keep pushing for 10 seconds and rest for 6. Repeat the exercise for 5 minutes. From repetition to repetition, the intensity with which you push on the chair can be varied. Within any given repetition, the intensity may also vary from start to finish.

**Attention:** If this exercise causes pain, mainly in the shoulders, reduce the amount of force being used. If the pain does not disappear completely, it is better to stop.

## 27  Pole back

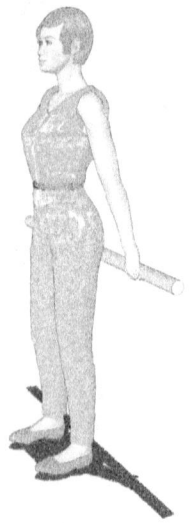

When working the shoulder muscles to offset imbalances, do not forget to do exercises that tone the muscles that permit your arms to move back. To do this, a workout using a slight amount of resistance may be helpful.

**Initial position:** Stand with a pole (such as a broomstick) grasped behind you, with both arms totally straight and near the body. The palms of your hands should be facing away from you.

**Workout:** Slowly lift the pole away from your body as far back as possible. Return to the resting position without moving your back. Repeat this for 3 to 5 minutes. If you feel fatigued after a while, you can stop, do another exercise, and return to complete the remaining time.

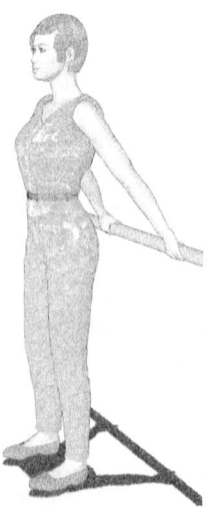

**Attention:** Even though you might be able to move one arm farther than the other, the movement should be symmetrical. Once this exercise can be done comfortably, you can add weight to the pole (between 2 and 10 lbs).

## 28 Back to the wall

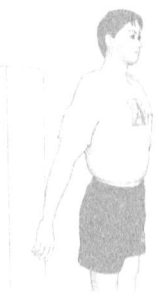

Isometric-type exercises may be helpful for working out your shoulder muscles. These are less likely to tear the tendons and are particularly useful for musicians who have pain in this area.

**Initial position:** Stand with your back to a wall, about 8-16 inches (20–40 cm) away from it. Your spinal column should be straight, taking care not to increase the curve of the back (avoid *hyperlordosis*). Place the palm of the hand of the arm being exercised on the wall.

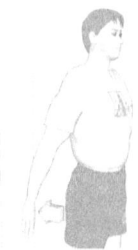

**Workout:** Press your hand against the wall for 6 seconds then rest for 6-10 seconds. Repeat 15 times. From repetition to repetition, the intensity with which you press your hand can be varied. Within any given repetition, the intensity may also vary from start to finish.

**Attention:** Your shoulder should not move forward when exerting pressure against the wall. The distance to the wall should vary from day to day.

## 29 Pectoral to the wall

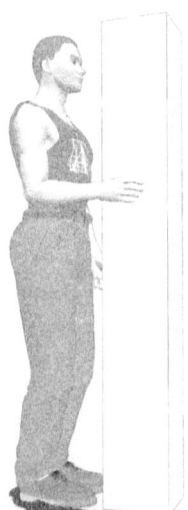

This is an exercise similar to the one done seated in the chair. Its objective is to tone the muscles used to lower the shoulder.

**Initial position:** Stand perpendicular to a door frame or in a corner, with your feet firmly planted on the ground, back straight and the hand of the side being exercised touching the wall with your palm. You can *bend your elbow* 90° or fully *extend* it.

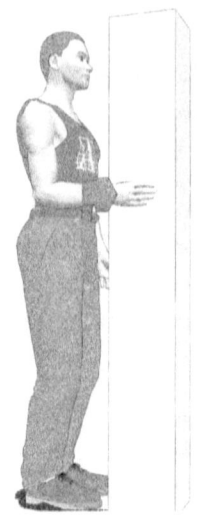

**Workout:** Press your hand against the wall for 6 seconds then rest for 6 seconds. Repeat 15 times. From repetition to repetition, the intensity with which you press your hand can be varied. Within any given repetition, the intensity may also vary from start to finish.

**Attention:** Every now and then, change the position of your elbow. You can exercise with any elbow angle between 90° and full *extension*. If you wish, both arms can be worked simultaneously.

## 30  Back with elastic band

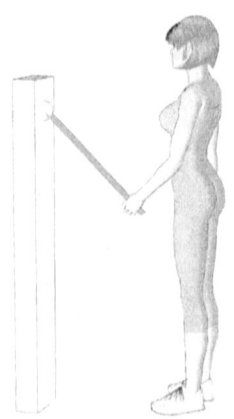

A workout with elastic bands is helpful for compensating imbalances experienced by musicians in their shoulders and backs.

**Initial position:** An elastic band (or similar device) that can be tied to a door knob (or similar object) is required. Once tied, grab the elastic band by the other end. Stand facing the object on which the elastic band was tied with both feet planted flat on the ground, back straight, at a distance where the elastic band is slightly in tension.

# CHAPTER THREE

## EXERCISES BY REGION OF THE BODY

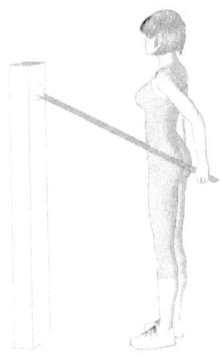

**Workout:** Pull the elastic band moving your hand back as much as your arm and the elastic band allow. The pace should be 2-3 seconds for the movement back and 2-3 seconds for the return, keeping the tension of the elastic band constant. Repeat this around 20 times (for a total of 2 minutes). It is not necessary to pull the elastic band back in a perfectly straight line. Each repetition can have a different path as well as sinusoidal movements within the repetition. The tension of the band can also be changed by standing closer or farther from the point where the band is attached.

**Attention:** You should not feel any pain. Do not pull the band all the way back if doing so causes pain..

## 31  Pectoral elastic band

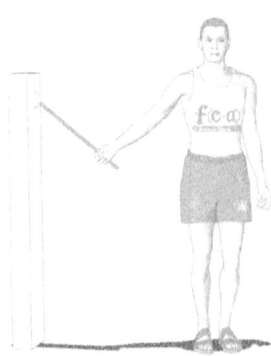

To fully tone your shoulder, exercise *30-Back with elastic band* should be done along with this pectoral exercise.

**Initial position:** An elastic band (or similar device) that can be tied to a door knob (or similar object) is required. Once tied, grab the elastic band by the other end. Stand sideways to the object on which the elastic band was tied with both feet planted flat on the ground, back straight, at a distance where the elastic band is slightly in tension and your arm is laterally separated from your body (*abduction*).

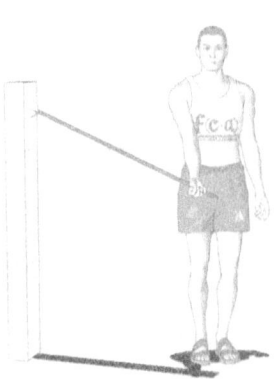

**Workout:** Pull the exercise band inward, moving your hand in front of your body, as if you wanted to touch your hip on the opposite side. Keep your *elbow extended*. The pace should be 2-3 seconds for the inward movement and 2-3 seconds for the return, keeping the tension of the elastic band constant. Repeat this around 20 times (for a total of 2 minutes). It is not necessary to pull the elastic band in a perfectly straight line. Each repetition can have a different path as well as sinusoidal movements within the repetition. The tension of the band can also be changed by standing closer or further from the point where the band is attached.

**Attention:** You should not feel any pain. Do not pull the band all the way if doing so causes pain.

# CHAPTER THREE

EXERCISES BY REGION OF THE BODY

# NECK AND DORSAL REGION OF THE BACK

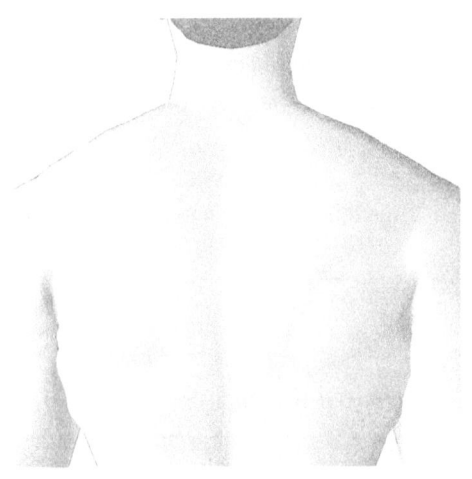

The area around the spinal column is extremely sensitive to tension, both from physical and psychological causes. Furthermore, while playing a musical instrument or during daily activities (e.g., when working at the computer), musicians tend to hunch the shoulders, thereby generating continuous and unnecessary tension in this zone. This tension leads to unwanted *muscle contractions*, which can cause discomfort and limit the fluidity of arm and hand movements.

The muscles in this zone are already in constant use, mainly to support posture. Musicians rarely need to work on strengthening them except in special cases.

Accordingly, the workout in this area should be focused on flexibility and stretching exercises, without the need for specific toning exercises.

## FLEXIBILITY EXERCISES

*19-Raising and lowering the shoulders*, in addition to being helpful for shoulder flexibility, is also a flexibility exercise for the neck and upper back areas. The following exercises are also recommended:

### 32  Yes with the neck

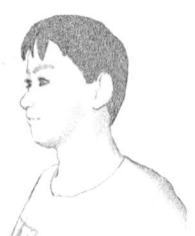

The front and back muscles of the neck (*trapezius*[34], *splenius*[32], *sternocleidomastoid*[33], etc.) are the ones that generally accumulate the most tension when playing an instrument. Flexibility exercises prepare you to withstand this tension.

**Initial position:** Stand or sit with your feet firmly planted on the ground, your back as straight as possible and your arms relaxed at your sides or on your thighs.

**IN TUNE**

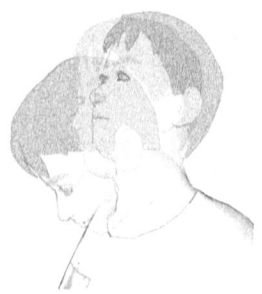

**Workout:** Slowly lower your head until your chin is on your chest then start the movement in the opposite direction. You should not reach the maximum upward *extension* since this could be harmful for the spinal column. A good guide for the correct amount of *extension* will be going just to the point where, without moving your eyes, you start to see the ceiling above your head. Repeat 10 times.

**Attention:** It is of the utmost importance not to attempt the maximum upward *extension* nor to move too quickly.

## 33  Maybe with the neck

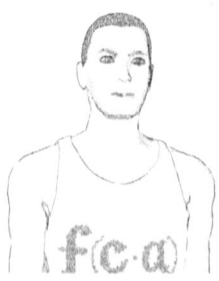

It is important to work your neck in a *tilting* motion. This type of movement is generally not done symmetrically while playing an instrument and, therefore, needs to be counterbalanced.

**Initial position:** Stand or sit with your arms resting on your legs or hanging at your sides and your head facing forward.

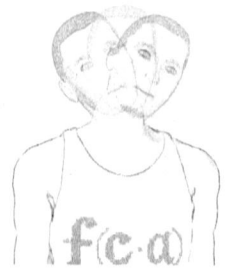

**Workout:** Slowly *tilt your head* as far as possible to one side, bringing your ear to your shoulder; then start the movement in the opposite direction. Repeat 10 times.

**Attention:** Try not to raise your shoulders as this reduces mobility and diminishes the efficacy of the exercise. Always keep your head facing forward. In these and other exercises involving the neck, creaking or popping sounds might be noticed and should be considered normal so long as they do not cause pain.

### 34  No with the neck

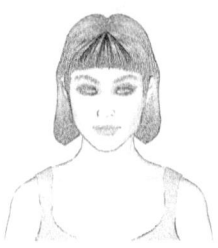

As with the other exercises that work this area, neck rotations make it possible to work on mobility and to prepare for playing at the same time.

**Initial position:** Sit or stand with your arms resting on your legs or hanging at your sides and your head facing forward.

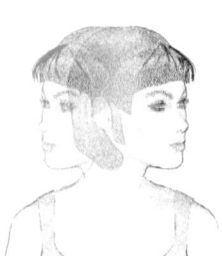

**Workout:** Slowly turn your neck (*rotation*) as far as possible so that your chin is over your shoulder; then start the movement in the opposite direction. Repeat 10 times.

**Attention:** Always keep your eyes straight ahead.

## STRETCHING EXERCISES

### 35  Back of the neck

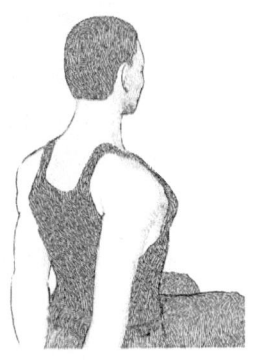

The *splenius*[32], located on the nape of the neck, tends to accumulate stress and become contracted along with the other muscles that maintain the neck's posture. This should be counterbalanced with stretching exercises.

**Initial position:** Stand with your legs slightly apart, or comfortably seated. Clasp your wrist behind your back with the opposite arm of the side you want to stretch.

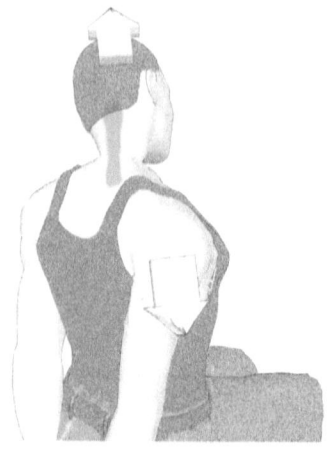

**Stretch:** *Tilt your head* down (*flexion of the neck*) and in the opposite direction of the side that you want to stretch. Pull your arm down to lower the shoulder. The greater the *flexion of the neck*, the more the *splenius*[32] will be stretched. Hold the stretch for 20 seconds per side.

**Attention:** It is important to not raise your shoulder. If seated, an option is to grasp the leg of the chair with the hand of the side you wish to stretch leaving your other arm free. You can then utilize your free arm by raising it above your head, placing your hand on your ear, and pulling your head down to make the stretch more intense.

## 36  Front of the neck

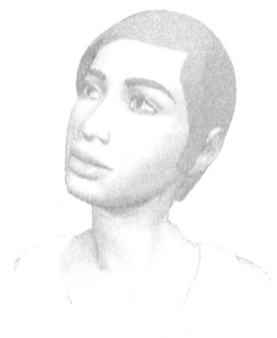

The *sternocleidomastoid*[33] is one of the most important muscles in the front of the neck. It maintains posture, moves the head, and has a tendency to contract when used. This stretch helps avoid the tendency to contract.

**Initial position:** For stretching the right side: Sitting or standing, *tilt your head* to the left (raising your right ear toward the ceiling), *extend your neck* and *rotate* slightly toward the right.

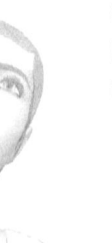

**Stretch:** For stretching the right side: Lift your chin up by rotating your head toward the left. Hold the stretch for 20 seconds per side.

# CHAPTER THREE

**EXERCISES BY REGION OF THE BODY**

**Attention:** Relax your shoulders and do not pull your head too far back when raising your chin.

## 37 Side of the neck

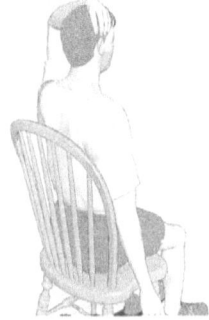

The upper part of the *trapezius*[32] is one of the areas of the back that most tends to accumulate stress in musicians. Therefore, it will be one of the zones of your body that needs to receive the most attention when stretching.

**Initial position:** Sit or stand with your legs slightly apart. On the side you want to stretch, let your arm hang down with your shoulder fully relaxed. Drape your opposite arm over your head and grasp near your ear.

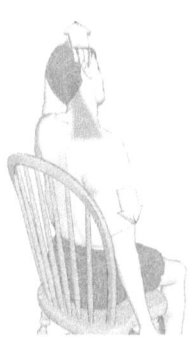

**Stretch:** *Tilt your neck* opposite the side you want to stretch, helping with the hand on your head. Lower the shoulder on the side being stretched as much as possible. Hold the stretch for 20 seconds per side.

**Attention:** Perform this stretch slowly and be aware of the onset of any discomfort in the spinal column. If your notice any discomfort, slightly *flex* or *extend* your neck to find a point where there is no pain.

## 38 Scapula levator

Together with the *trapezius*[32], the *scapula levator*[29], which is a muscle that connects the neck and the shoulder blade, is one of the muscles that often tenses up in musicians. That is why adding this stretch to your workout routine is crucial for staying in good shape.

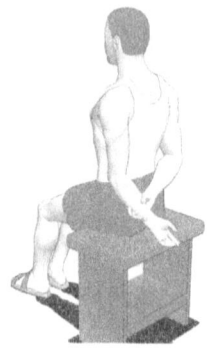

**Initial position:** Sit or stand with your legs slightly apart. Keep the shoulder on the side you want to stretch relaxed and low.

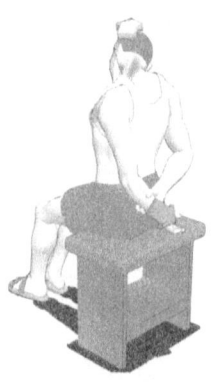

**Stretch:** *Tilt your head* opposite the side you want to stretch and then *flex your neck* forward. You can use your other arm to help lower your shoulder by grasping the wrist of the side you want to stretch behind your back and pulling down. Hold the stretch for 20 seconds per side.

**Attention:** By increasing or decreasing the degree of *flexion in the neck*, the area where you feel the stretch can be modified. This allows you to maximize the stretch of this region.

## 39 Interscapular

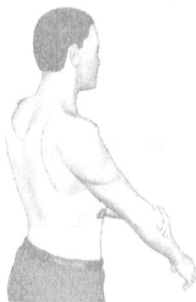

It is the *rhomboid muscles*[27] that make it possible to pull back your shoulders. Playing an instrument generally stresses these muscles so it is necessary to counterbalance with this stretch.

**Initial position:** Stand with your legs slightly apart. Put an arm in front of you and grasp your elbow with your opposite hand. Try grasping behind your elbow or in front on your forearm and decide which is better for you.

| CHAPTER THREE | EXERCISES BY REGION OF THE BODY |

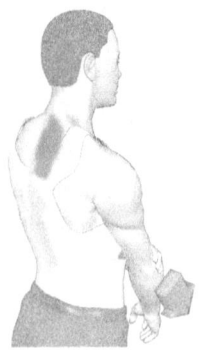

**Stretch:** Using the arm that is grasping your forward arm, pull your shoulder forward and inward. Hold the stretch for 20 seconds per side.

**Attention:** Since the *rhomboid muscles*[27] connect your shoulder blades, it is crucial to stretch the shoulder toward the front of your body. This will not be possible if the muscles are not completely relaxed. Although you can grasp your arm wherever you like, the stretch is easiest if you grasp right above the elbow.

## TONING EXERCISES

Musicians generally have a well-toned neck and back (thoracic region) as a result of playing their instrument. Moreover, since these muscles are generally tense or contracted when playing, a strengthening workout can be counterproductive if it does not take the need for recovery into account.

Musicians do not need to tone the muscles in this area, except in specific cases of previous injury. In that instance, consult with a medical professional who is knowledgeable about your type of injury and your playing requirements. This professional can design a proper strengthening regime for you.

# LUMBAR AND ABDOMINALS

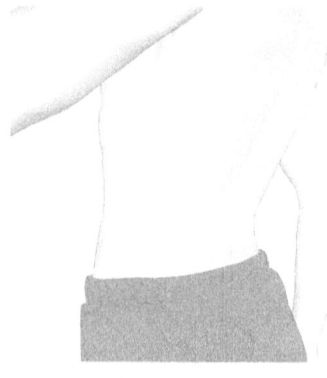

The lumbar region (lower back) can be problematic since it is affected, either directly or indirectly, by bad posture, asymmetrical use, and stresses created by most musical instruments.

The same is true for the cervical and dorsal areas (neck and upper back). Since they involve muscles that control posture (tonic muslces), it is generally not necessary for musicians to strengthen these muscles. The exercises for these areas focus exclusively on flexibility and stretching to achieve greater freedom of movement and better postural control.

On the other hand, the abdominal muscles in the front part of the abdomen, as opposed to the tonic (postural) muscles of the back, do not need stretching but rather increased toning. Strong abdominal muscles make it possible to more easily adopt proper spinal posture and provide good breath control.

For this reason, the focus for this zone of the body will be exclusively on toning within a maintenance program. You should recall that all toning exercises should not be performed directly before or after playing.

## FLEXIBILITY EXERCISES

The exercise *20-Twisting the chest and arms* aids flexibility of the upper part of the body as well as the lumbar and abdominal areas. The following flexibility exercises are also recommended for this area:

### 40  Flexing the lumbar spine

The lower part of the spine, the lumbar zone, is where most stress is generally concentrated. This stress is accentuated in people who have bad posture and those who have to maintain a certain position for long periods of time or play in an imbalanced manner, as frequently happens with musicians. The lumbar zone should be prepared so it can better support these stresses.

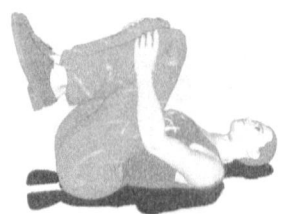

**Initial position:** Lie down face up on a firm surface. Bring both legs toward your chest. Grasp your legs by the knees.

| CHAPTER THREE | EXERCISES BY REGION OF THE BODY |

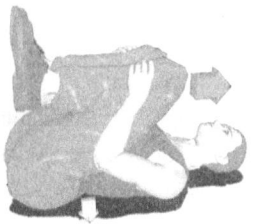

**Workout:** Bring your knees to your chest. Pull with your hands to *straighten the lumbar curve*. Hold this position for 20 seconds, and repeat at least twice.

**Attention:** Try to gradually increase the degree of movement, without bouncing. Do not let any part of the shoulders rise from the ground.

## 41 Child's pose

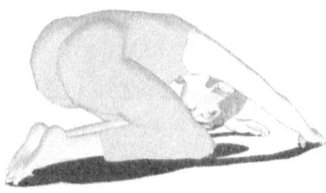

This exercise achieves flexibility and stretching for an important part of the back muscles. Therefore, it is highly recommended for musicians.

**Initial position:** Kneel on the ground with your hands and arms stretched out in front of your head and your forehead facing the ground. The *gluteus maximus*[10] muscles are in contact with your calves and your head in line with the spinal column.

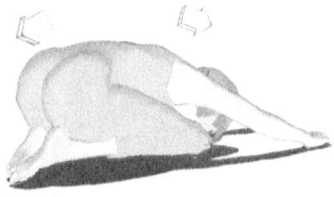

**Workout:** The intention is to expand your back by trying to reach as far as possible with your hands, walking them in front of your body, but without lifting the buttocks from your legs. Hold this position for 20 seconds, and repeat at least twice.

**Attention:** Do not raise your head or lift your *gluteus maximus*[10] from your legs while this exercise is being performed.

## 42 Straightening the lumbar curve on the ground

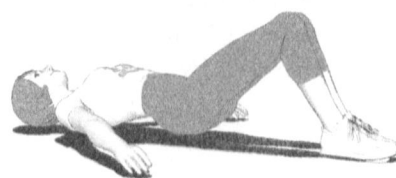

Maintaining the proper lumbar curvature (the lower part of your spinal column) is a key component for comfortable posture. This exercise improves control of this area.

**Initial position:** Lie down, face up, with your *knees bent* and feet flat on the ground.

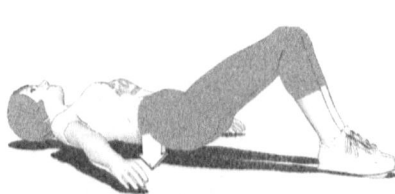

**Workout:** Breathe in and hold for 3 to 5 seconds. While you are holding your breath, place your entire back in contact with the ground. You should try to raise your navel up and in (*straightening the lumbar curve*) so that there is no space between the lumbar area and the ground. Start to exhale slowly while maintaining the position for a minimum of 10 seconds. Repeat 3 times.

**Attention:** Whenever the position of the exercise requires you to lie down with your face up, you should *bend your knees* in order not to strain your back. Never lift the sacrum from the ground.

## STRETCHING EXERCISES

### 43 Back

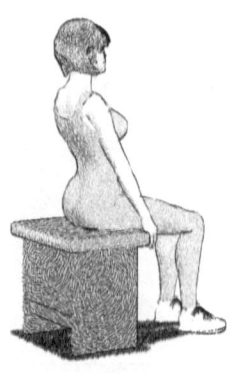

The muscles on both sides of the spinal column (*paravertebral muscles*[20]) are in continuous contraction to maintain your posture while you are playing. If properly stretched, they will better withstand stresses and be less prone to injury.

**Initial position:** Sit on a stool with your hands by your side, legs slightly apart, and feet on the floor.

# CHAPTER THREE

**EXERCISES BY REGION OF THE BODY**

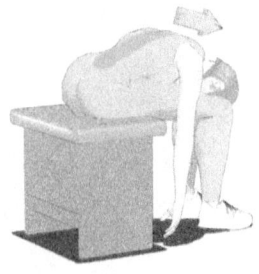

**Stretch:** Let your body fall forward and down, with your hands outside of your legs. Arch your entire back from the neck. Place your head between your legs to increase the stretch. Maintain this position for 20 seconds.

**Attention:** Let your shoulders fall forward to help stretch the thoracic region.

## 44 Lateral abdominal muscles

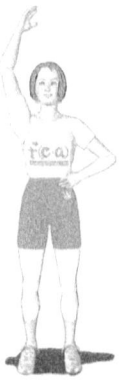

The *obliques*[17] generally work in a very limited motion. Stretching them helps make up for this.

**Initial position:** Stand with your feet slightly apart. Place one arm over your head and the hand of your other arm resting on your waist.

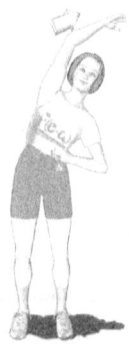

**Stretch:** Bend at your waist towards the side of your resting arm. Keep the other arm straight above your head. Hold the stretch for 20 seconds per side.

**Attention:** Although this stretch is mostly achieved by reaching your arm upward, you can perform the exercise without raising your arm if you have shoulder problems. Do not excessively bend the waist to the side since this can injure the spinal column.

## 45 Lower back

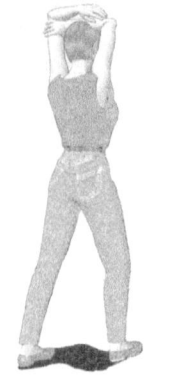

The *quadratus lumborum*[23] helps maintain good posture in the lower part of the spine. This stretch keeps it toned.

**Initial position:** Stand with one leg forward and your *knee slightly bent*. Keep your back leg stretched with your feet facing forward and your weight evenly balanced on both feet. On the same side as your back foot, lift your elbow until you can touch your ear with the inner part of your arm. With your opposite hand, grasp your arm from behind near your elbow.

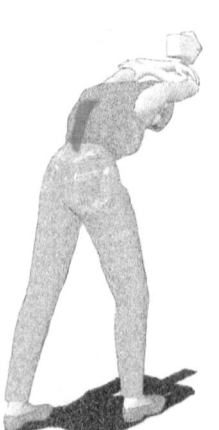

**Stretch:** Lift your elbow up to indirectly stretch your ribs. Then roll the upper part of your back over your chest while pulling your elbow towards your front foot. Hold the stretch for 20 seconds per side.

**Attention:** Do not press down or support your arms on your head or your neck. Always keep pulling on your elbow.

## 46 Spinal twist

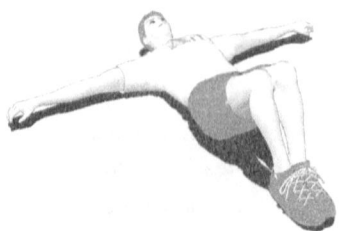

This stretch exercises not only a good number of the back and abdominal muscles but also the joints of the spinal column. It is therefore highly recommended.

**Initial position:** Lie down face up with your *knees bent*, feet planted on the ground, and your arms outward in the shape of a cross.

# CHAPTER THREE

**EXERCISES BY REGION OF THE BODY**

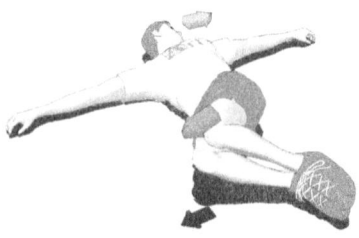

**Stretch:** Let your knees fall to one side without raising your shoulders off the ground. Turn your head to the side opposite your legs. Try to touch the ground with your ear. Hold the stretch for 20 seconds per side.

**Attention:** Remember that stretches are based on feelings. Accordingly, the level of twist must be sufficient to cause a pleasant stretching feeling. The 20-second holding time is also a guideline. You may hold this stretch longer if you think your back needs it or if it is pleasurable to do so.

## 47 Front hip area

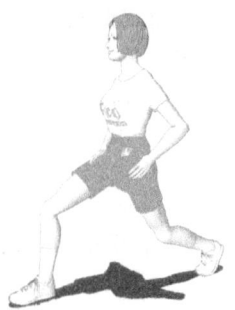

The *iliopsoas*[12] is not visible from the outside since it is located inside the belly towards the back, yet it plays a very important role in the posture of the back. It is therefore crucial to stretch it in your workout even though you may not be able to identify it.

**Initial position:** Stand with your *knees slightly bent* and place one leg forward and one leg back. The heel of the back leg should be off the ground. Try to *straighten the lumbar curve* as much as possible.

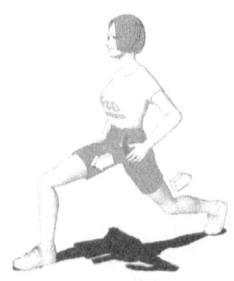

**Stretch:** Lower your body *bending the knee* of your forward leg, as if you were trying to bend it beyond your foot. To increase the tension, stretch your back leg by *extending the knee*. Hold the stretch for 20 seconds per side.

**Attention:** Your back (spinal column) should at all times be straight and immobile. It is recommended that you do this stretch near a wall or object where you can support yourself to better maintain your balance.

## TONING EXERCISES

### 48 Rectus abdominals

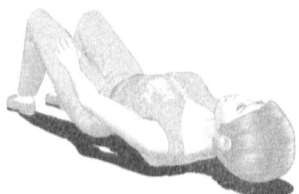

Toning the abdominal muscles is crucial to prevent problems with the spinal column. However, many abdominal exercises can be harmful for musicians. A method of exercising called irradiation (compound movements that indirectly work a given muscle) is safe for the *rectus abdominis*[26].

**Initial position:** Lie down face up with both legs together and *knees bent*. For the leg you want to work, *bend the hip* and *knee* 90°. Place your hand on the knee or thigh of the bent leg.

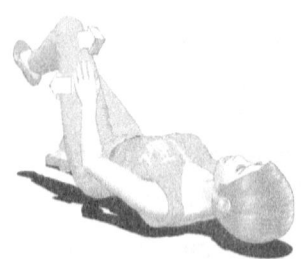

**Workout:** Bring your leg towards your chest while pressing your hand firmly against your leg. Your goal is to have equal pressure between the pushing of your hand and the lifting of your leg so that neither one succeeds in pushing the other and no movement is generated. Maintain this push/pull equilibrium for 6 seconds. Repeat this at least 10 times per leg. It is recommended to be done up to 20 times per leg.

**Attention:** Whenever the position of the exercise requires you to lie down with your face up, you should *bend your knees* in order not to strain your back. Never lift the sacrum from the ground.

### 49 Oblique abdominals

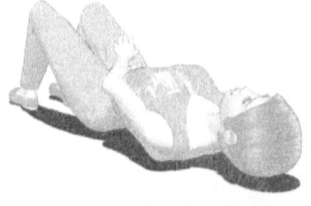

The *obliques*[17] should also be exercised to help stabilize your spinal column. This is also an irradiation exercise (indirectly rather than directly exercising the abdominals) and will be performed using levers created between your arm and leg.

**Initial position:** Lying down, face up, with your *knees bent*. For the leg you want to work, *bend the hip* and *knee* 90°. Place your hand from the opposite side in contact with your thigh or knee.

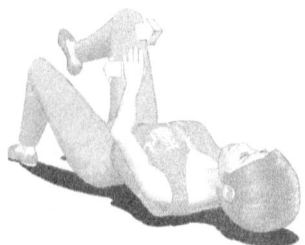

**Workout:** Bring your leg towards your chest while pressing your hand firmly against your leg. Your goal is to have equal pressure between the pushing of your hand and the lifting of your leg so that neither one succeeds in pushing the other and no movement is generated. Maintain this push/pull equilibrium for 6 seconds. Repeat this at least 10 times per leg. It is recommended to be done up to 20 times per leg.

**Attention:** Whenever the position of the exercise requires you to lie down, face up, you should *bend your hip* and *knees* in order not to strain your back.

## 50 Abdominal workout using a wall

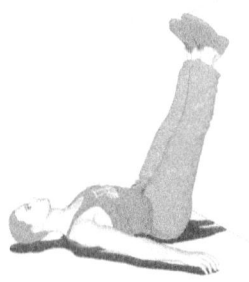

Another way of working the abdominal muscles without harming the spinal column is by using a wall, as shown in this exercise.

**Initial position:** Lie down face up with your feet together and up on a wall. The distance between the wall and the lower part of your back must be 8-16 inches (20-40 cm). The shorter the distance, the less work the abdominal muscles will do. However, exercising too far away from the wall might put too much stress on the lumbar area (*quadratus lumborum*[23]). You should experiment to find the distance that best suits you.

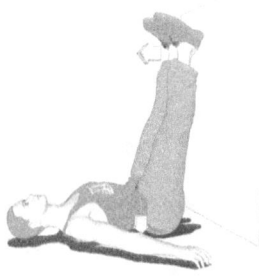

**Workout:** A) Bring your feet out from the wall 1 - 2 inches (2 to 3 cm) and hold that position for 10 seconds. Repeat 6 times. B) Then bring your feet out from the wall 1 - 2 inches (2 to 3 cm) and slightly rock your feet side to side (about 30° to each side). It is recommended that this exercise be done for at least 10 seconds and repeated 6 times. C) Finally, bring your feet out from the wall 1 - 2 inches (2 to 3 cm) and do a scissor movement (alternate crossing one leg over the other). It is recommended that this exercise be done for at least 10 seconds and repeated 6 times.

**Attention:** Although the legs should be kept more or less vertical, the angle of the hips with respect to the wall can vary. Your lumbar spine, however, should never arch when you bring your feet out from the wall. The farther the feet are away from the wall, the more your lumbar spine is likely to arch.

## 51 Hamstrings and abdominals

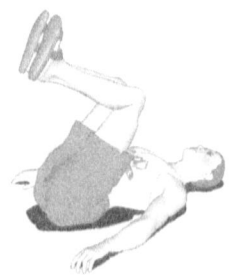

This exercise promotes the toning of the abdominal muscles along with the stretching of the *hamstring muscles*[11] (the muscles of the back part of the thigh). Since both muscle groups are involved in the position of the spinal column and how it works, this combination is worthy of attention.

**Initial position:** Lie down face up and bring both legs toward your chest. Keep your hands on the floor by your sides.

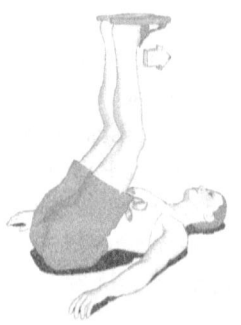

**Workout:** Maintaining the angle of *flexion in the hip*, extend your knees as much as possible, adding *extension of your ankles*. Repeat a minimum of 6 times holding the position for at least 10 seconds.

**Attention:** Do not reduce the angle of your hips when moving your legs. Remember, since this is a floor exercise and you are face up, *bend your hips* and *knees* to prevent strain on the back. The more flexible you are, the more you will be able to *extend your knees*.

# CHAPTER THREE

EXERCISES BY REGION OF THE BODY

# THIGH AND LEG

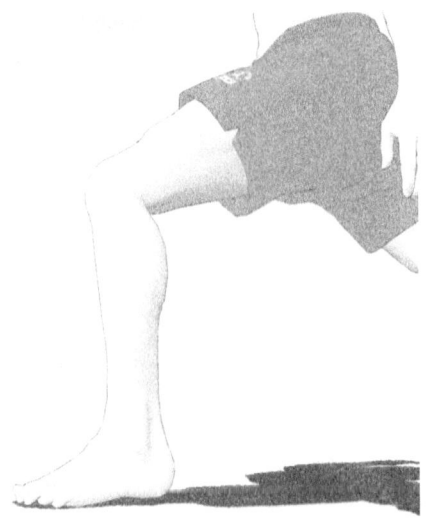

Even though most musicians may not use their legs for playing their instrument, exercising the thighs is recommended for posture control of the pelvis and the spinal column.

As this essentially involves a group of tonic (postural) muscles that are highly prone to contraction over the years, musicians should definitely incorporate stretching exercises of this area in their maintenance program.

## FLEXIBILITY EXERCISES

For musicians, the stretching exercises shown below are also helpful for flexibility of the thigh and leg. Therefore, flexibility and stretching for this area will be covered using the same exercises.

## STRETCHING EXERCISES

**52  Leg back 1**

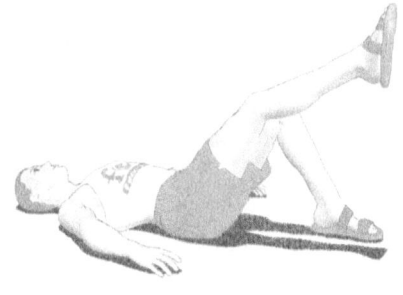

The *hamstring muscles*[11] are the main muscles of the back part of the thigh. If they are not stretched regularly, they will gradually shorten and have repercussions on your back and posture.

**Initial position:** Lie down face up with one leg *bent at the knee* and foot flat on the ground. The other leg should be somewhat *bent at the knee* but raised off the ground. Place your hands at your sides while keeping your head on the ground without increasing cervical curvature in the neck.

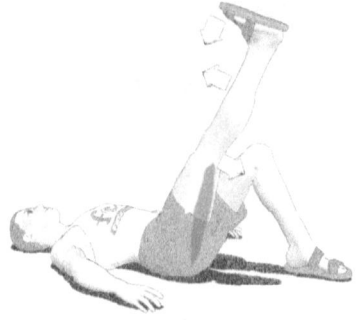

**Stretch:** Raise your leg while completely *extending your knee* and *ankle*. Hold the stretch 20 seconds per leg and, as it involves a large muscle, repeat 2 or 3 times.

**Attention:** If your head is in a strained or uncomfortable position, put a thin cushioning material (a folded towel, a small pillow, etc.) beneath your head.

## 53  Leg back 2

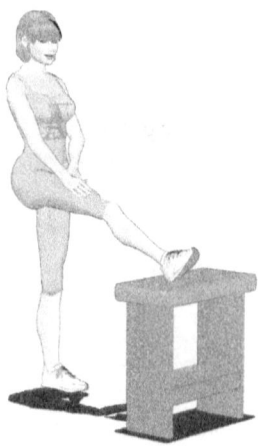

Although the *hamstring muscles*[11] are located in the back part of your leg, they modify the position of your pelvis, which affects the curves of your back. Stretching these muscles regularly improves the overall health of the spinal column.

**Initial position:** Stand, keeping your back straight at all times. With one foot on the ground, place the back of the heel of your other foot out in front of you on a stool, table, etc. This leg should have the *knee only slightly bent*. The more elastic your rear leg muscles are, the higher the stool can be.

# CHAPTER THREE

## EXERCISES BY REGION OF THE BODY

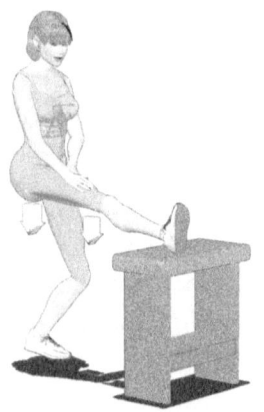

**Stretch:** *Bend the knee* of the leg on the ground, thus lowering your body and increasing the *extension of the knee* of the leg on the stool. If you want to increase the intensity of the stretch, move your torso forward from the pelvis *straightening the lumbar curve* and thoracic region. Hold the stretch for 20 seconds per leg. Repeat 2 or 3 times since it involves large muscles.

**Attention:** The stool should be fairly high; otherwise, the knee of the leg on which you are standing may bend too much and cause strain. To avoid losing your balance, hold on to a wall or the back of a chair.

## 54 Glutes

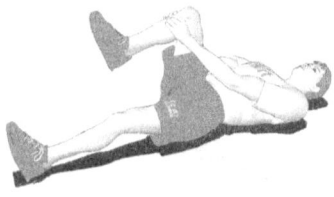

The gluteal area contains several muscles, the most important being the *gluteus maximus*[10]. They help move the hip and assist in maintaining the position of the pelvis, leg, and back. This stretch makes it possible to exercise them properly.

**Initial position:** Lie down face up with one leg stretched out and the other *bent at the knee*. Grasp the leg that is bent with your arms.

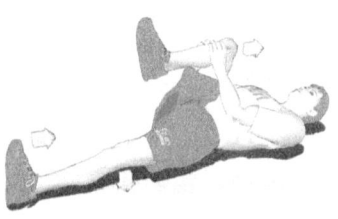

**Stretch:** Bring your knee to your chest. Keep your other leg flat on the ground, fully extended, with your toes pointing up towards your head (full *extension of the ankle*). Hold the stretch for 20 seconds per leg. Repeat 2 or 3 times since it is a large muscle.

## 55 Internal leg 1

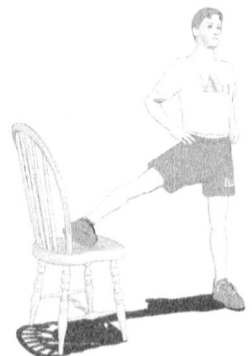

The group of *adductor*[1] muscles can be worked in various ways. Keeping these muscles elastic can prevent the pelvic area from becoming overly stressed.

**Initial position:** Place a chair at your side. Stand next to the chair, with your back straight and your arms at your sides or on your waist. Put one foot on the chair with the inside of the foot on the seat of the chair and your toes pointed forward. Stand up straight on your other leg.

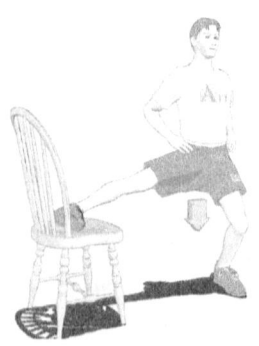

**Stretch:** Try to lower the hip of the leg that is being stretched, without tilting, by *bending your opposite knee*. Hold the stretch for 20 seconds per side. Repeat 2 or 3 times as this involves a large muscle.

**Attention:** Choose the height of the chair or stool based on how flexible you are; the more elasticity you have, the higher your chair or stool can be. The intensity of the stretch can be increased by bringing your chest forward to *straighten the lumbar curve* and thoracic region. If you have knee problems, do not do this stretch and replace with *56-Internal leg 2*.

## 56 Internal leg 2

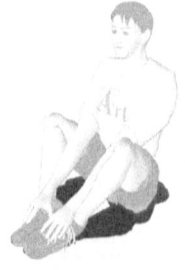

The *adductors*[1] can also be exercised while you are seated on the ground. This way both sides can be worked at the same time.

**Initial position:** Sit on the ground with your *knees bent*. Touch the soles of your feet together close to your body, and *straighten the lumbar curve*.

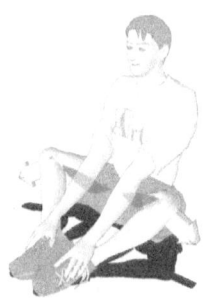

**Stretch:** Separate your knees (lowering them to the ground) without separating your feet or arching your back. Hold the stretch for 20 seconds. Since it involves a large muscle, repeat 2 or 3 times.

**Attention:** The stretch can be increased by using your elbows to push down on your legs.

## 57 Front leg

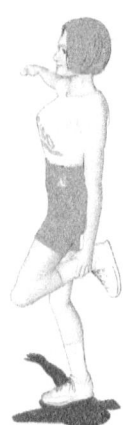

The *quadricep*[24] is a powerful muscle that, among other things, helps you maintain your posture when you are standing. It should be stretched regularly to maintain sufficient elasticity.

**Initial position:** Stand on one leg and grab the other leg from behind near your ankle. Without separating one leg from the other, bring your heel close to your *gluteus maximus*[10]. Keep your back straight and do not increase the lumbar curvature (avoid *hyperlordosis*). You may hold onto a wall or chair for balance with the hand you are not using.

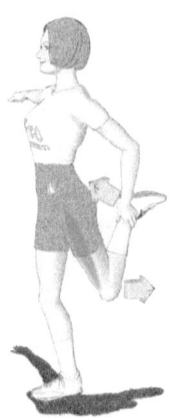

**Stretch:** With your hand holding your ankle, push your thigh back while keeping your *knee bent*. Hold the stretch for 20 seconds on each leg. Since it involves a large muscle, repeat 2 or 3 times.

**Attention:** Do not arch your back or tilt your body forward.

## 58 Calf muscles

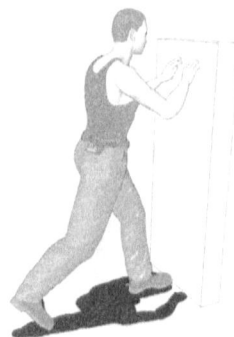

The *triceps surae*[36] makes up the main part of the calf. It is attached to the heel by the Achilles tendon. This muscle can become overstressed and experience small ruptures if the accumulated tension is not counterbalanced by properly stretching.

**Initial position:** Stand with your hands on a wall, with one leg forward and the other back with your *knees slightly bent*.

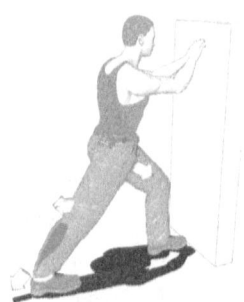

**Stretch:** Move your pelvic area (waist) forward to the wall, while the knee of your back leg is stretched. Try to keep your back foot flat on the ground. Hold the stretch for 20 seconds per leg. Since this involves a large muscle, repeat 2 or 3 times.

**Attention:** The feet should always face forward; do not arch your spinal column (avoid *hyperlordosis*). The distance from your feet to the wall is one of the factors that will determine the degree of stretching. Accordingly, stand close to the wall if the calf is stiff.

## TONING EXERCISES

It is not necessary for musicians to tone this area.

# CHAPTER THREE
### EXERCISES BY REGION OF THE BODY

# FACE

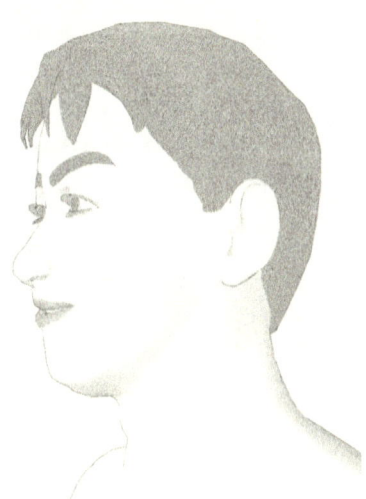

The muscles that help shape the mouth are extremely delicate and are not solidly anchored to bone. Some muscles connect directly to other muscles, thereby constituting a type of muscular grid.

In the playing of wind instruments, these muscles are often prone to high stresses. Accordingly, if this area is not properly exercised, there can easily be problems leading to reduced performance ability.

To avoid injuries and to maintain a high performance level of the facial muscles, it is recommended to do a thorough warm-up (flexibility and stretching exercises) and cool-down (stretches), as well as toning exercises without the instrument.

## FLEXIBILITY EXERCISES

### 59 Vowels and Consonants

It is necessary to consciously prepare the delicate muscles that make up the mouth and allow you to play. Doing so requires making broad movements that work as many of the mimic muscles (those that belong to the face) as possible. This exercise is one example, but other similar movements are equally worthwhile.

**Initial position:** Stand or sit with your feet firmly planted on the ground. Totally relax the muscles of the face, neck and shoulders. Analyze the level of relaxation zone by zone (forehead, cheeks, cheekbones, tongue, etc.).

# IN TUNE

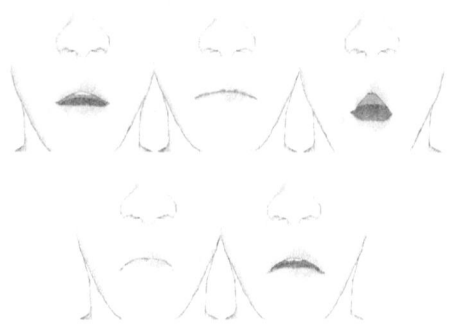

**Workout:** This involves moving the muscles around the mouth area. One possibility is to do a succession of vowels and consonants (for example A-M-O-P-E) exaggerating the articulation. You can also simulate chewing gum with your mouth open, exaggerating the movements.

**Attention:** People who have temporomandibular joint problems (TMJ) should try to do broad movements of the lips without overly separating the teeth.

## STRETCHING EXERCISES

### 60 One-sided face stretch

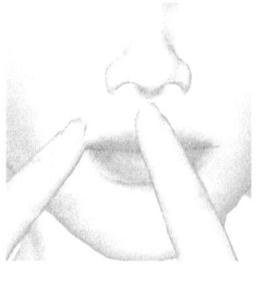

The *orbicularis oris muscle*[18] is a delicate structure that is not designed to withstand stress when playing an instrument. This stretch prepares the muscle to deal with the stress as much as possible.

**Initial position:** Standing or seated, place the index finger of one hand on the center of the upper lip and the index finger of the other hand at the corner of your mouth where the upper lip joins the lower lip.

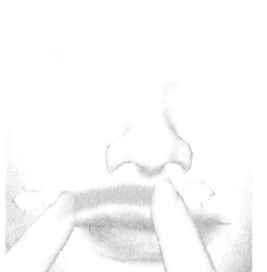

**Stretch:** Stretch the skin trying to move these two points away from each other (separate the two fingers). Hold the stretch for 20 seconds per side. Do the same with the lower lip.

# CHAPTER THREE

**EXERCISES BY REGION OF THE BODY**

**Attention:** As this is a very small set of muscles, you should be extra attentive to feelings in order to avoid injury. When stretching, you should try to differentiate any sensation felt in the skin from that of the muscle.

## 61 Two-sided face stretch

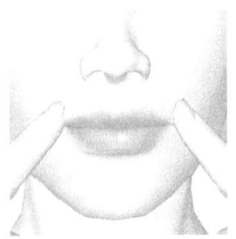

The *orbicularis oris muscle*[18] is not connected to the bones of the face. Being able to contract this muscle in an effective manner depends on the connections the muscles of the face have with each other. Therefore, a general stretch is desirable.

**Initial position:** Standing or seated, place your index fingers above the corners of your mouth on each side of your face.

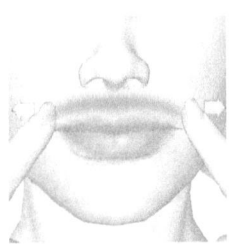

**Stretch:** Stretch the skin trying to move these two points away from each other (separate the two fingers). Hold the stretch for 20 seconds. Do the same with the lower lip.

**Attention:** Do not try to do both lips at the same time. First the upper lip and then the lower lip. As this is a very small set of muscles, you should be extra attentive to feelings in order to avoid injury. When stretching, you should try to differentiate any sensation felt in the skin from that of the muscle.

## TONING EXERCISES

### 62 Straight smile

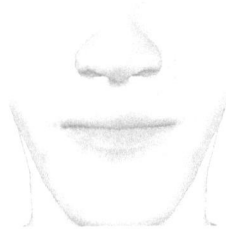

The muscles that form the embouchure are very delicate and are not designed to withstand a great deal of stress. For this reason, it is useful to keep these muscles toned with exercises that do not include the instrument.

**Initial position:** Sit or stand facing forward, making sure that all the muscles of the face are very relaxed.

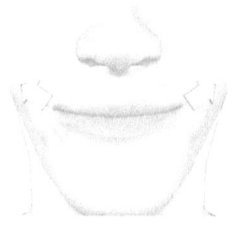

**Workout:** With the mouth in a straight line, try to pull the corners of the mouth with a certain intensity to the sides by means of the facial muscles. Hold the contraction 5-6 seconds and then relax for a similar period. Repeat a minimum of 5 times.

**Attention:** The first few times you do this exercise, it is recommended that you do it in front of a mirror to be sure that the exercise is being done properly and to avoid unnecessary tension in other muscles.

## 63 Sneer

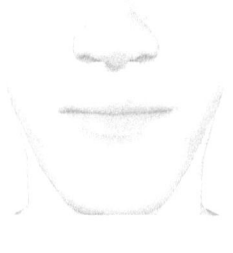

The musculature of the mouth, unlike most muscles, has no solid anchor point to the bone. Some muscles are connected to each other constituting a kind of muscular grid. This makes it difficult to properly exercise them, and more attention than usual should be devoted to their workout.

**Initial position:** Sit or stand facing forward, making sure that all the muscles of the face are relaxed.

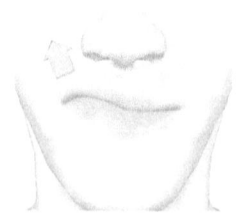

**Workout:** Try to raise one side of your mouth as if you were making a sneer. Maintain the contraction for 5 – 6 seconds and relax for an equal amount of time. Repeat a minimum of 5 times per side.

**Attention:** Be careful not to generate tension in other areas of the face or neck.

| CHAPTER THREE | EXERCISES BY REGION OF THE BODY |

## 64 Kiss

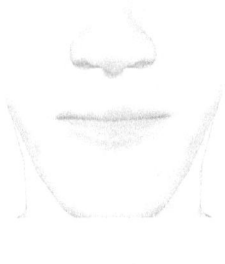

The *orbicularis oris muscle*[18] is the most important muscle for musicians who play wind instruments. It surrounds the entire opening of the mouth. This exercise makes it possible to isolate this muscle.

**Initial position:** Sit or stand facing forward, making sure that all the muscles of the face are relaxed.

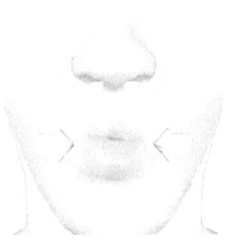

**Workout:** Bring the corners of your mouth together as if you wanted to kiss someone. Maintain the contraction for 5 – 6 seconds and relax for an equal amount of time. Repeat a minimum of 5 times.

**Attention:** Do not force your lips against your teeth.

## 65 Fish

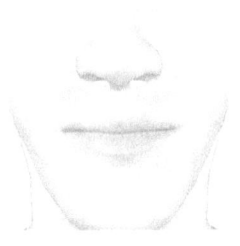

**Initial position:** Sit or stand facing forward, making sure that all the muscles of the face are relaxed.

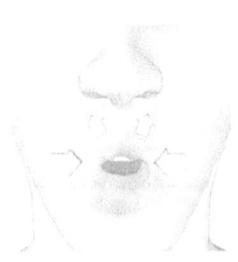

**Workout:** Bring the corners of your mouth together as if you wanted to kiss someone, but in this case do not close your lips completely. Reveal your teeth and gums like a fish. Maintain the contraction for 5 – 6 seconds and relax for an equal amount of time. Repeat a minimum of 5 times.

**Attention:** Pay special attention not to create tension in other areas of the face or neck.

## 66 Shivers

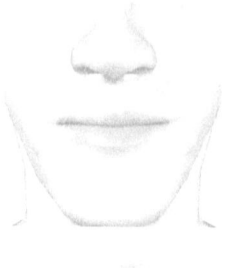

Your face muscles are also connected to the neck muscles. With this exercise both groups of muscles are worked together.

**Initial position:** Sit or stand facing forward, making sure that all the muscles of the face are relaxed.

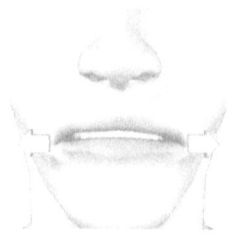

**Workout:** Direct your lower lip and the corners of your mouth down and out generating tension in the skin of the neck (shiver). Maintain the contraction 5 – 6 seconds and relax for an equal amount of time. Repeat a minimum of 5 times.

**Attention:** Some people are prone to cramping (painful involuntary contractions) in the muscles of the neck or below the tongue. If any of these exercises cause discomfort, reduce the intensity or skip such exercises entirely.

## 67 Upward smile

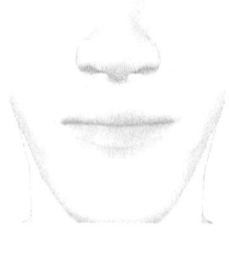

Each expression of the face implies the coordination of various muscles. A variety of exercises should be performed to involve the greatest number of these muscles.

**Initial position:** Sit or stand facing forward, making sure that all the muscles of the face are relaxed.

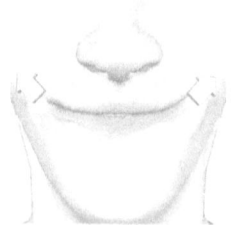

**Workout:** Raise the corners of the mouth as if you were going to smile. Maintain the contraction 5 – 6 seconds and relax for an equal amount of time. Repeat a minimum of 5 times.

**Attention:** Pay special attention to not generate tension in other areas of the face or neck.

## 68 Frown

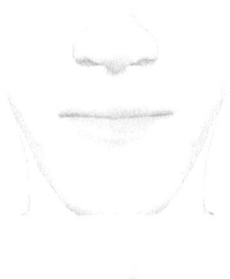

Trying to exercise specific parts of the face not only tones the muscles but also makes them more effective and improves your coordination.

**Initial position:** Sit or stand facing forward, making sure that all the muscles of the face are relaxed.

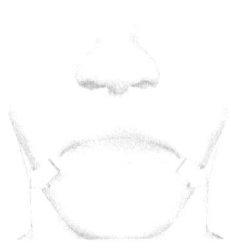

**Workout:** With your teeth slightly together, pull the corners of your mouth back with a simultaneous drop of the lower lip (frown). Maintain the contraction 5 – 6 seconds and relax for an equal amount of time. Repeat a minimum of 5 times.

**Attention:** Pay special attention to not generate tension in other areas of the face or neck.

Chapter Four

# EXERCISES BY INSTRUMENT

Even though all musicians generally use similar muscle groups, it is necessary to establish certain differences in the way each instrumentalist exercises due to the variations of instruments regarding their shape, dimensions, way they are held, technical requirements, and the physical stresses that they involve.

Based on analysis of the zones that are the most strained and those that have the greatest tendency to accumulate stresses, a set of exercises has been selected for each group of instruments. Two basic situations have been considered: before playing (warm-up) and after playing (cool-down).

The goal of the warm-up exercises are to prepare the joints, muscles, tendons, nervous system, etc. for playing while preventing injuries and improving performance.

The cool-down exercises help restore equilibrium, possibly altered by musical activity, and promote the recovery process.

In order to be more efficient, instruments sharing similar physical demands have been grouped together even though they are physically dissimilar or from an entirely separate instrumental family.

Look for your instrument in the list on pages 91-95 to determine your group, or refer to the picture on page 90 to find the playing posture of your instrument.

Recommended exercises have been proposed for before and after playing for each of the groups. In both situations, there is a choice between an essential program (for those who want a routine that contains the most important exercises, which should never be skipped) and a complete program (for those who have more time and wish to work all areas thoroughly).

Exercises indicated as "optional" are those that, while useful and recommended for the given instrument, are the least important. If you have limited time and must skip any exercises, these are the ones that can be skipped.

To promote ease of use, each exercise is delineated by name, number, and suggested duration or repetition. Also included is an image of the exercise and the page(s) where

**CHAPTER FOUR**                        **EXERCISES BY INSTRUMENT**

a detailed explanation can be found. Remember these exercises should be done on both sides of the body (right and left) and it is recommended to start on the side that will be subject, or has been subject, to higher stress loads.

As already mentioned, these programs must be accompanied by meaningful practice on the instrument. This should include specific warm-ups and cool-downs (a gradual increase in the intensity and difficulty when starting to play and a gradual decrease at the end of the session), a break every 20-40 minutes (during which you can stretch the most strained areas), appropriate posture, regulation of the physical elements (height of the chair, distance and height of the music stand, etc.), and the right environmental conditions (light, temperature, humidity, and noise).

It is also advisable to introduce variation into your practice routines. Try changing up the order of the exercises or using different exercises that work the same areas. You can also do the routines at different times of the day, in different locations, or even using different chairs or different instruments if applicable, etc.

# IN TUNE

## EXERCISES GROUPED BY PLAYING POSITIONS

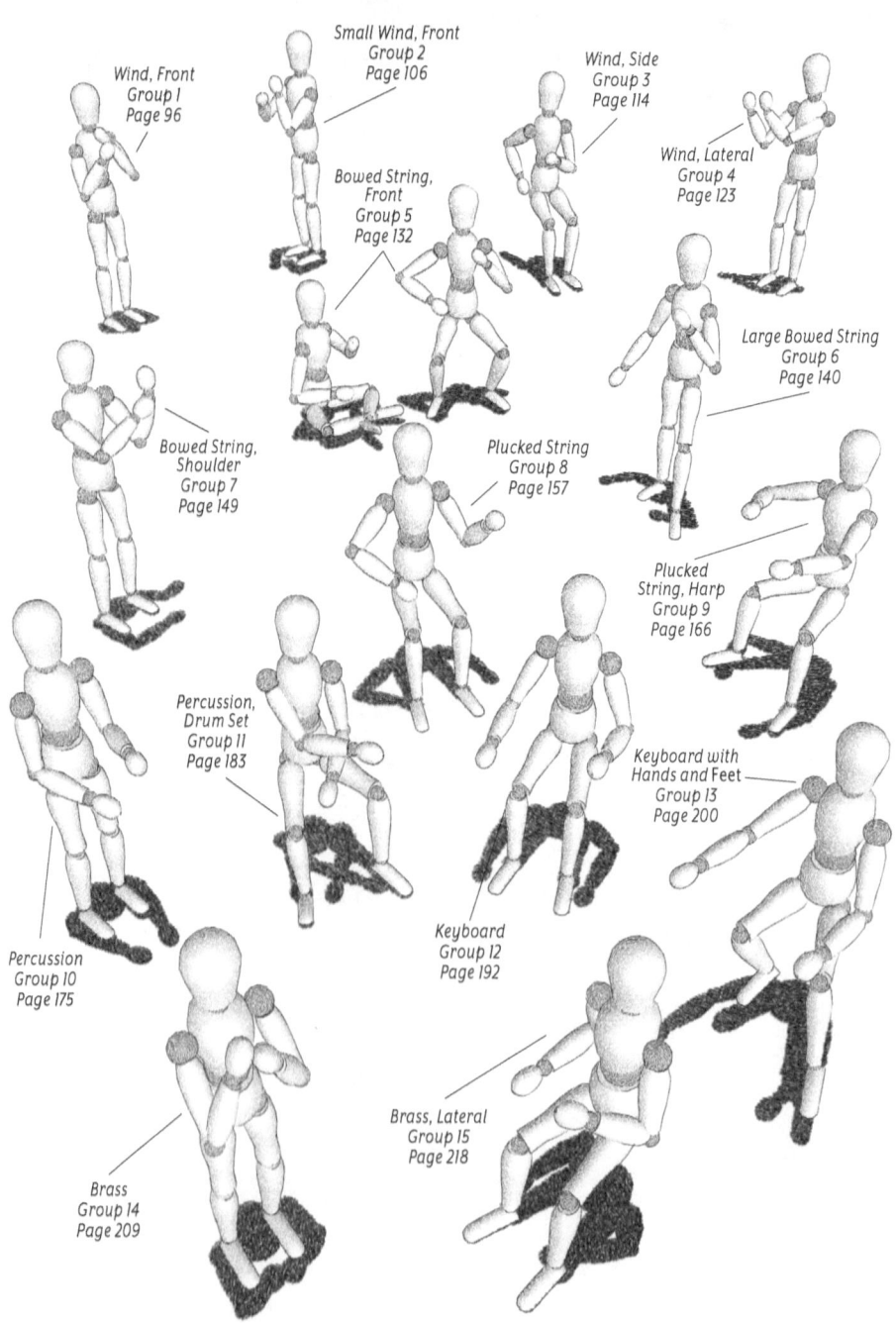

90

CHAPTER FOUR                                        EXERCISES BY INSTRUMENT

# INSTRUMENTS BY GROUP

## A

| | |
|---|---|
| Accordion | *Group 12* |
| Algaita | *Group 1* |

## B

| | |
|---|---|
| Bagpipes | *Group 1* |
| Balalaika | *Group 8* |
| Bamboo scraper | *Group 10* |
| Bandoneon | *Group 12* |
| Banjo | *Group 8* |
| Baritone Horn | *Group 15* |
| Bass, double (stand up) | *Group 6* |
| Bass drum | *Group 10* |
| Bass, electric (guitar) | *Group 8* |
| Bassoon | *Group 3* |
| Bombard | *Group 1* |
| Bongos | *Group 10* |
| Bonang | *Group 10* |
| Bouzouki | *Group 8* |
| Bugle | *Group 14* |

## C

| | |
|---|---|
| Castanets | *Group 10* |
| Celeste | *Group 12* |
| Cello | *Group 5* |
| Chalice drum | *Group 10* |
| Chalumeau | *Group 1* |
| Charango | *Group 8* |
| Chirimía | *Group 1* |
| Chitarrone | *Group 8* |
| Cimbalom | *Group 10* |
| Clarinet | *Group 1* |
| Clarinet, alto | *Group 1* |
| Clarinet, bass | *Group 1* |
| Clarinet, contrabass | *Group 1* |
| Clarinet, Eb | *Group 2* |
| Clavichord | *Group 12* |
| Clavicymbalum | *Group 12* |
| Clavicytherium | *Group 12* |
| Concertina | *Group 12* |
| Congas | *Group 10* |
| Contrabassoon | *Group 1* |
| Cornet | *Group 14* |
| Cornetto | *Group 1* |

# INSTRUMENTS BY GROUP

## C, continued

| | |
|---|---|
| Crotales | *Group 10* |
| Cymbals | *Group 10* |

## D

| | |
|---|---|
| Darbuka | *Group 10* |
| Debuka | *Group 10* |
| Deduk | *Group 1* |
| Didgeridoo | *Group 14* |
| Djembe | *Group 10* |
| Doumbek | *Group 10* |
| Drum set | *Group 11* |
| Drums | *Group 10* |
| Dulcian | *Group 3* |
| Dulcimer | *Group 10* |
| Dulzaina | *Group 1* |
| Dumbec | *Group 10* |
| Dumbelek | *Group 10* |
| Dumbeg | *Group 10* |

## E

| | |
|---|---|
| English horn | *Group 1* |
| Erhu | *Group 5* |
| Euphonium | *Group 15* |

## F

| | |
|---|---|
| Flabiol | *Group 2* |
| Flageolet | *Group 2* |
| Flugelhorn | *Group 14* |
| Flute | *Group 4* |
| Frame drum | *Group 10* |
| French horn | *Group 15* |

## G

| | |
|---|---|
| Gendèr | *Group 10* |
| Glockenspiel | *Group 10* |
| Goblet drum | *Group 10* |
| Gralla | *Group 1* |
| Güiro | *Group 10* |
| Guitar, electric | *Group 8* |
| Guitar, acoustic | *Group 8* |
| Guitarron (Mariachi guitar) | *Group 8* |

CHAPTER FOUR                                    EXERCISES BY INSTRUMENT

# INSTRUMENTS BY GROUP

## H

| Hardenger | Group 7 |
| Harmonica | Group 2 |
| Harp | Group 9 |
| Harpsichord | Group 12 |
| Heckelphone | Group 1 |
| Helicon | Group 15 |
| Hichiriki | Group 2 |

## K

| Kemence | Group 5 |
| Kena/Quena | Group 2 |

## L

| Lute | Group 8 |

## M

| Mandolin | Group 8 |
| Maracas | Group 10 |
| Marimba | Group 10 |
| Melodica | Group 2 |
| Mellophone | Group 14 |
| Metallophone | Group 10 |

## N

| Ney | Group 2 |

## O

| Oboe | Group 1 |
| Oboe d'amore | Group 1 |
| Organ | Group 13 |
| Organ, portable | Group 12 |
| Organ, pump | Group 13 |
| Organetto | Group 12 |
| Ottavino | Group 12 |
| Oud | Group 8 |

## P

| Pan flute | Group 14 |
| Piano | Group 12 |
| Piccolo | Group 4 |
| Pungi (snake charmer) | Group 2 |

## R

| Raita | Group 1 |
| Ratchet | Group 10 |
| Rebab | Group 5 |
| Rebec | Group 7 |

## INSTRUMENTS BY GROUP

### R, continued

| | |
|---|---|
| Recorder | Group 1 |

### S

| | |
|---|---|
| Sackbut, alto | Group 14 |
| Sackbut, bass | Group 14 |
| Sackbut, contrabass | Group 14 |
| Sackbut, tenor | Group 14 |
| Sarrusophone | Group 1 |
| Sarangi | Group 5 |
| Saxophone, alto | Group 3 |
| Saxophone, baritone | Group 3 |
| Saxophone, bass | Group 3 |
| Saxophone, sopranino (straight & curved) | Group 1 |
| Saxophone, soprano (straight & curved) | Group 1 |
| Saxophone, tenor | Group 3 |
| Shawm, alto | Group 1 |
| Shawm, catalan | Group 1 |
| Shehnai | Group 1 |
| Silbote (basque flute) | Group 2 |
| Sitar | Group 8 |
| Snare drum | Group 10 |

### S, continued

| | |
|---|---|
| Suona | Group 1 |
| Sousaphone | Group 15 |
| Spinet | Group 12 |

### T

| | |
|---|---|
| Tablah | Group 10 |
| Talking drum | Group 10 |
| Tambourine | Group 10 |
| Tanbur | Group 8 |
| Tar | Group 8 |
| Tarabuka | Group 10 |
| Tarota | Group 1 |
| Temple block | Group 10 |
| Tenor horn | Group 14 |
| Tenor tuba | Group 15 |
| Thearbo | Group 8 |
| Tibetan horn | Group 14 |
| Timpani | Group 10 |
| Toumperleki | Group 10 |
| Triangle | Group 10 |
| Trombone, alto | Group 14 |
| Trombone, bass | Group 14 |

## INSTRUMENTS BY GROUP

### T, continued

| | |
|---|---|
| Trombone, contrabass | *Group 14* |
| Trombone, tenor | *Group 14* |
| Trombone, valve | *Group 14* |
| Trumpet | *Group 14* |
| Trumpet, Piccolo | *Group 14* |
| Tuba | *Group 15* |
| Tubular bells | *Group 10* |
| Txistu (basque flute) | *Group 2* |

### U

| | |
|---|---|
| Uilleann pipes | *Group 9* |
| Ukulele | *Group 8* |

### V

| | |
|---|---|
| Veena | *Group 6* |
| Vibraphone | *Group 10* |
| Viola | *Group 7* |
| Viola d'amore | *Group 7* |

### V, continued

| | |
|---|---|
| Viola da gamba | *Group 5* |
| Viola da braccio | *Group 7* |
| Violin | *Group 7* |
| Virginals | *Group 12* |

### W

| | |
|---|---|
| Whip | *Group 10* |
| Woodblock | *Group 10* |

### X

| | |
|---|---|
| Xylophone | *Group 10* |

### Z

| | |
|---|---|
| Zither | *Group 8* |
| Zurna | *Group 1* |

IN TUNE

# GROUP 1
# WIND, FRONT

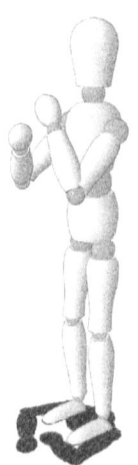

This group of wind instruments generally has weight that is primarily supported by the thumbs as well as arms that must be kept in a raised position that *closes the shoulders* and increases *dorsal hunching*.

In addition to certain mouth exercises, it is crucial for the work-out program to include exercises to counterbalance the stresses in the aforementioned areas.

## BEFORE PLAYING

**Essential**
9 minutes 30 seconds in total; 7 minutes without optional exercises

| | | | |
|---|---|---|---|
| 1 | | Finger mobility 1<br>10 times (optional) | Page 29 |
| 12 | | Full arm rotations<br>10 times (optional) | Page 38 |
| 32 | | Yes with the neck<br>10 times (optional) | Page 57 |
| 33 | | Maybe with the neck<br>10 times (optional) | Page 58 |

**CHAPTER FOUR**                                              **EXERCISES BY INSTRUMENT**

| # | | Exercise | Page |
|---|---|---|---|
| 34 | | No with the neck<br>10 times (optional) | Page 59 |
| 37 | | Side of the neck<br>20" + 20" | Page 61 |
| 38 | | Scapula levator<br>20" + 20" | Page 61 |
| 35 | | Back of the neck<br>20" + 20" (optional) | Page 59 |
| 36 | | Front of the neck<br>20" + 20" | Page 60 |
| 15 | | Fist in<br>20" + 20" | Page 41 |
| 17 | | Hand down<br>20" + 20" | Page 42 |
| 59 | | Vowels and consonants<br>30" | Page 79 |

**IN TUNE**

| 61 | | Two-sided face stretch<br>20" + 20" | Page 81 |
|---|---|---|---|
| 21 | | Chest<br>20" + 20" | Page 47 |
| 44 | | Lateral abdominal muscles<br>20" + 20" | Page 67 |
| 5 | | Thumb down<br>20" + 20" | Page 32 |
| 6 | | Thumb back<br>20" + 20" | Page 33 |

**Complete**
14 minutes 10 seconds in total; 9 minutes 40 seconds without optional exercises

| 1 | | Finger mobility 1<br>10 times | Page 29 |
|---|---|---|---|
| 2 | | Finger mobility 2<br>10 times (optional) | Page 30 |

# CHAPTER FOUR

**EXERCISES BY INSTRUMENT**

| 19 | | Raising and lowering the shoulders<br>10 times (optional) | Page 46 |
|---|---|---|---|
| 12 | | Full arm rotations<br>10 times (optional) | Page 38 |
| 20 | | Twisting the chest and arms<br>10 times | Page 46 |
| 32 | | Yes with the neck<br>10 times (optional) | Page 57 |
| 33 | | Maybe with the neck<br>10 times (optional) | Page 58 |
| 34 | | No with the neck<br>10 times | Page 59 |
| 37 | | Side of the neck<br>20" + 20" | Page 61 |
| 38 | | Scapula levator<br>20" + 20" | Page 61 |

| 35 | | Back of the neck<br>20" + 20" (optional) | Page 59 |
|---|---|---|---|
| 36 | | Front of the neck<br>20" + 20" | Page 60 |
| 14 | | Fist out<br>20" + 20" | Page 40 |
| 16 | | Hand back<br>20" + 20" | Page 42 |
| 59 | | Vowels and consonants<br>30" | Page 79 |
| 60 | | One-sided face stretch<br>20" + 20" + 20" +20" | Page 80 |
| 61 | | Two-sided face stretch<br>20" + 20" (optional) | Page 81 |
| 21 | | Chest<br>20" + 20" | Page 47 |

| | | | |
|---|---|---|---|
| CHAPTER FOUR | | | EXERCISES BY INSTRUMENT |

| | | | |
|---|---|---|---|
| 44 | | Lateral abdominal muscles<br>20" + 20" | Page 67 |
| 5 | | Thumb down<br>20" + 20" | Page 32 |
| 6 | | Thumb back<br>20" + 20" | Page 33 |
| 3 | | Hand muscles<br>20" + 20" + 20" + 20" (optional) | Page 31 |
| 4 | | Palm of the hand<br>20" | Page 31 |
| 43 | | Back<br>20" | Page 66 |

## AFTER PLAYING

**Essential**
7 minutes 20 seconds in total; 6 minutes without optional exercises

| | | | |
|---|---|---|---|
| 37 | | Side of the neck<br>20" + 20" | Page 61 |

**IN TUNE**

| 38 | | Scapula levator<br>20" + 20" | Page 61 |
|---|---|---|---|
| 35 | | Back of the neck<br>20" + 20" (optional) | Page 59 |
| 36 | | Front of the neck<br>20" + 20" | Page 60 |
| 15 | | Fist in<br>20" + 20" | Page 41 |
| 17 | | Hand down<br>20" + 20" | Page 42 |
| 61 | | Two-sided face stretch<br>20" + 20" | Page 81 |
| 21 | | Chest<br>20" + 20" | Page 47 |
| 44 | | Lateral abdominal muscles<br>20" + 20" | Page 67 |

# CHAPTER FOUR  EXERCISES BY INSTRUMENT

| 5 | | Thumb down<br>20" + 20" | Page 32 |
|---|---|---|---|
| 6 | | Thumb back<br>20" + 20" (optional) | Page 33 |

## Complete
10 minutes 40 seconds in total; 8 minutes without optional exercises

| 37 | | Side of the neck<br>20" + 20" | Page 61 |
|---|---|---|---|
| 38 | | Scapula levator<br>20" + 20" | Page 61 |
| 35 | | Back of the neck<br>20" + 20" (optional) | Page 59 |
| 36 | | Front of the neck<br>20" + 20" | Page 60 |
| 14 | | Fist out<br>20" + 20" | Page 40 |

**IN TUNE**

| | | | |
|---|---|---|---|
| 16 | | Hand back<br>20" + 20" | Page 42 |
| 60 | | One-sided face stretch<br>20" + 20" + 20" + 20" | Page 80 |
| 61 | | Two-sided face stretch<br>20" + 20" (optional) | Page 81 |
| 21 | | Chest<br>20" + 20" | Page 47 |
| 44 | | Lateral abdominal muscles<br>20" + 20" | Page 67 |
| 5 | | Thumb down<br>20" + 20" | Page 32 |
| 6 | | Thumb back<br>20" + 20" | Page 33 |
| 3 | | Hand muscles<br>20" + 20" + 20" + 20" (optional) | Page 31 |

| CHAPTER FOUR | | | EXERCISES BY INSTRUMENT |
|---|---|---|---|
| 4 | | Palm of the hand<br>20" | Page 31 |
| 43 | | Back<br>20" | Page 66 |

IN TUNE

# GROUP 2
# SMALL WIND, FRONT

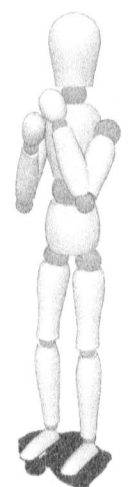

Despite the advantage of these instruments being lightweight, their small dimensions can result in finger strain and excessive *bending of the elbows*. In addition, these musicians need to keep the arms raised in a position that *closes the shoulders* and increases *dorsal hunching*.

This makes it necessary for these musicians to do specific exercises, within this program, that compensate for these stresses.

## BEFORE PLAYING

**Essential**
(8 minutes 20 seconds in total; 4 minutes 50 seconds without optional exercises)

| | | | |
|---|---|---|---|
| 1 | | Finger mobility I<br>10 times (optional) | Page 29 |
| 12 | | Full arm rotations<br>10 times (optional) | Page 38 |
| 32 | | Yes with the neck<br>10 times (optional) | Page 57 |
| 33 | | Maybe with the neck<br>10 times (optional) | Page 58 |

# CHAPTER FOUR

**EXERCISES BY INSTRUMENT**

| | | | |
|---|---|---|---|
| 34 | | No with the neck<br>10 times (optional) | Page 59 |
| 37 | | Side of the neck<br>20" + 20" | Page 61 |
| 38 | | Scapula levator<br>20" + 20" | Page 61 |
| 35 | | Back of the neck<br>20" + 20" (optional) | Page 59 |
| 36 | | Front of the neck<br>20" + 20" | Page 60 |
| 15 | | Fist in<br>20" + 20" | Page 41 |
| 17 | | Hand down<br>20" + 20" | Page 42 |
| 59 | | Vowels and consonants<br>30" | Page 79 |

# IN TUNE

| 61 | 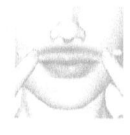 | Two-sided face stretch<br>20" + 20" | Page 81 |
|---|---|---|---|
| 3 | 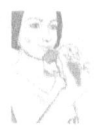 | Hand muscles<br>20" + 20" + 20" + 20" (optional) | Page 31 |
| 4 | 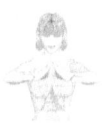 | Palm of the hand<br>20" | Page 31 |

## Complete
(13 minutes 10 seconds in total; 8 minutes without optional exercises)

| 1 | 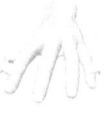 | Finger mobility 1<br>10 times | Page 29 |
|---|---|---|---|
| 2 | 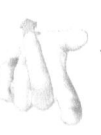 | Finger mobility 2<br>10 times (optional) | Page 30 |
| 19 | 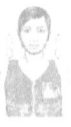 | Raising and lowering the shoulders<br>10 times (optional) | Page 46 |
| 12 | 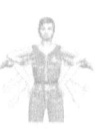 | Full arm rotations<br>10 times | Page 38 |

**CHAPTER FOUR**                        **EXERCISES BY INSTRUMENT**

| 20 | Twisting the chest and arms<br>10 times (optional) | Page 46 |
|---|---|---|
| 32 | Yes with the neck<br>10 times (optional) | Page 57 |
| 33 | Maybe with the neck<br>10 times (optional) | Page 58 |
| 34 | No with the neck<br>10 times | Page 59 |
| 37 | Side of the neck<br>20" + 20" | Page 61 |
| 38 | Scapula levator<br>20" + 20" | Page 61 |
| 35 | Back of the neck<br>20" + 20" (optional) | Page 59 |
| 36 | Front of the neck<br>20" + 20" | Page 60 |

| | | | |
|---|---|---|---|
| 14 | | Fist out<br>20" + 20" | Page 40 |
| 17 | | Hand down<br>20" + 20" | Page 42 |
| 59 | | Vowels and consonants<br>30" | Page 79 |
| 60 | | One-sided face stretch<br>20" + 20" + 20" + 20" | Page 80 |
| 61 | | Two-sided face stretch<br>20" + 20" (optional) | Page 81 |
| 3 | | Hand muscles<br>20" + 20" + 20" + 20" (optional) | Page 31 |
| 4 | | Palm of the hand<br>20" | Page 31 |
| 39 | | Interscapular<br>20" + 20" | Page 62 |

| CHAPTER FOUR | | | EXERCISES BY INSTRUMENT |

| 23 | 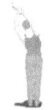 | Latissimus dorsi<br>20" + 20" | Page 49 |

## AFTER PLAYING

**Essential**
(6 minutes 20 seconds in total; 4 minutes 20 seconds without optional exercises)

| 37 | | Side of the neck<br>20" + 20" | Page 61 |

| 38 | | Scapula levator<br>20" + 20" | Page 61 |

| 35 | | Back of the neck<br>20" + 20" (optional) | Page 59 |

| 36 | | Front of the neck<br>20" + 20" | Page 60 |

| 14 | | Fist out<br>20" + 20" | Page 40 |

| 16 | | Hand back<br>20" + 20" | Page 42 |

# IN TUNE

| 61 | | Two-sided face stretch  
20" + 20" | Page 81 |

| 3 | | Hand muscles  
20" + 20" + 20" + 20" (optional) | Page 31 |

| 4 | | Palm of the hand  
20" | Page 31 |

## Complete
(9 minutes in total; 6 minutes 20 seconds without optional exercises)

| 37 | | Side of the neck  
20" + 20" | Page 61 |

| 38 | | Scapula levator  
20" + 20" | Page 61 |

| 35 | | Back of the neck  
20" + 20" (optional) | Page 59 |

| 36 | | Front of the neck  
20" + 20" | Page 61 |

**CHAPTER FOUR**                                                **EXERCISES BY INSTRUMENT**

| No. | | Exercise | Page |
|---|---|---|---|
| 14 | | Fist out<br>20" + 20" | Page 40 |
| 16 | | Hand back<br>20" + 20" | Page 42 |
| 60 | | One-sided face stretch<br>20" + 20" + 20" + 20" | Page 80 |
| 61 | | Two-sided face stretch<br>20" + 20" (optional) | Page 81 |
| 3 | | Hand muscles<br>20" + 20" + 20" + 20" (optional) | Page 31 |
| 4 | | Palm of the hand<br>20" | Page 31 |
| 39 | | Interscapular<br>20" + 20" | Page 62 |

# IN TUNE

# GROUP 3
# WIND, SIDE

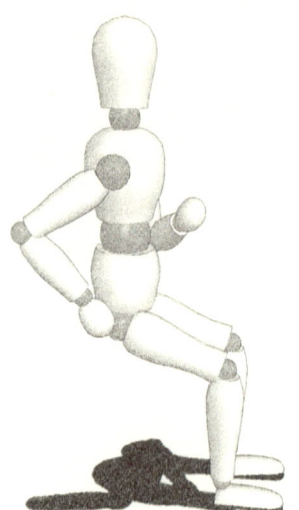

The primary characteristics of this group involve instruments of significant weight, which must be played in a clearly asymmetrical position, with a twisting of the torso and a possible compromise of the shoulder.

In addition to the specific mouth exercises, it is important for the work-out program to include exercises that counterbalance these physical strains.

## BEFORE PLAYING

**Essential**
(8 minutes 10 seconds in total; 6 minutes without optional exercises)

| 1 | | Finger mobility 1<br>10 times (optional) | Page 29 |
|---|---|---|---|
| 12 | | Full arm rotations<br>10 times (optional) | Page 38 |
| 32 | | Yes with the neck<br>10 times (optional) | Page 57 |
| 33 | | Maybe with the neck<br>10 times (optional) | Page 58 |

# CHAPTER FOUR — EXERCISES BY INSTRUMENT

| 34 | No with the neck<br>10 times (optional) | Page 59 |
|---|---|---|
| 37 | Side of the neck<br>20" + 20" | Page 61 |
| 38 | Scapula levator<br>20" + 20" | Page 61 |
| 35 | Back of the neck<br>20" + 20" (optional) | Page 59 |
| 36 | Front of the neck<br>20" + 20" | Page 60 |
| 14 | Fist out<br>20" + 20" | Page 40 |
| 16 | Hand back<br>20" + 20" | Page 42 |
| 59 | Vowels and consonants<br>30" | Page 79 |

## IN TUNE

| 61 | | Two-sided face stretch<br>20" + 20" | Page 81 |
|---|---|---|---|
| 23 | | Latissimus dorsi<br>20" + 20" | Page 49 |
| 24 | | Rear shoulder<br>20" + 20" | Page 50 |

### Complete
(12 minutes 50 seconds in total; 9 minutes without optional exercises)

| 1 | | Finger mobility 1<br>10 times (optional) | Page 29 |
|---|---|---|---|
| 2 | | Finger mobility 2<br>10 times (optional) | Page 30 |
| 19 | | Raising and lowering the shoulders<br>10 times (optional) | Page 46 |
| 12 | | Full arm rotations<br>10 times (optional) | Page 38 |

# CHAPTER FOUR — EXERCISES BY INSTRUMENT

| | | | |
|---|---|---|---|
| 20 | | Twisting the chest and arms<br>10 times | Page 46 |
| 32 | | Yes with the neck<br>10 times (optional) | Page 57 |
| 33 | | Maybe with the neck<br>10 times (optional) | Page 58 |
| 34 | | No with the neck<br>10 times | Page 59 |
| 37 | | Side of the neck<br>20" + 20" | Page 61 |
| 38 | | Scapula levator<br>20" + 20" | Page 61 |
| 35 | | Back of the neck<br>20" + 20" (optional) | Page 59 |
| 36 | | Front of the neck<br>20" + 20" | Page 60 |

**IN TUNE**

| 15 | | Fist in<br>20" + 20" | Page 41 |
|---|---|---|---|
| 17 | | Hand down<br>20" + 20" | Page 42 |
| 59 | | Vowels and consonants<br>30" | Page 79 |
| 60 | | One-sided face stretch<br>20" + 20" + 20" + 20" | Page 80 |
| 61 | | Two-sided face stretch<br>20" + 20" (optional) | Page 81 |
| 23 | | Latissimus dorsi<br>20" + 20" | Page 49 |
| 24 | | Rear shoulder<br>20" + 20" | Page 50 |
| 4 | | Palm of the hand<br>20" | Page 31 |

| CHAPTER FOUR | | | EXERCISES BY INSTRUMENT |

| 39 | | Interscapular<br>20" + 20" | Page 62 |

| 43 | | Back<br>20" | Page 66 |

# AFTER PLAYING

**Essential**
(6 minutes in total; 5 minutes 20 seconds without optional exercises)

| 37 | | Side of the neck<br>20" + 20" | Page 61 |

| 38 | | Scapula levator<br>20" + 20" | Page 61 |

| 35 | | Side of the neck<br>20" + 20" (optional) | Page 59 |

| 36 | | Front of the neck<br>20" + 20" | Page 60 |

| 14 | | Fist out<br>20" + 20" | Page 40 |

# IN TUNE

| 17 | Hand down 20" + 20" | Page 42 |
| 61 | Two-sided face stretch 20" + 20" | Page 81 |
| 23 | Latissimus dorsi 20" + 20" | Page 49 |
| 24 | Rear shoulder 20" + 20" | Page 50 |

## Complete
(10 minutes in total; 7 minutes 20 seconds without optional exercises)

| 37 | Side of the neck 20" + 20" | Page 61 |
| 38 | Scapula levator 20" + 20" | Page 61 |
| 35 | Back of the neck 20" + 20" (optional) | Page 59 |

**CHAPTER FOUR**                                            **EXERCISES BY INSTRUMENT**

| 36 | | Front of the neck<br>20" + 20" | Page 60 |
|---|---|---|---|
| 14 | | Fist out<br>20" + 20" | Page 40 |
| 17 | | Hand down<br>20" + 20" | Page 42 |
| 60 | | One-sided face stretch<br>20" + 20" + 20" + 20" | Page 80 |
| 61 | | Two-sided face stretch<br>20" + 20" (optional) | Page 81 |
| 23 | | Latissimus dorsi<br>20" + 20" | Page 49 |
| 24 | | Rear shoulder<br>20" + 20" | Page 50 |
| 39 | | Interscapular<br>20" + 20" | Page 62 |

**IN TUNE**

| 43 | | Back<br>20" | Page 66 |
|---|---|---|---|

| 3 | | Hand muscles<br>20" + 20" + 20" + 20" (optional) | Page 31 |
|---|---|---|---|

| 4 | | Palm of the hand<br>20" | Page 31 |
|---|---|---|---|

CHAPTER FOUR                                    EXERCISES BY INSTRUMENT

# GROUP 4
# WIND, LATERAL

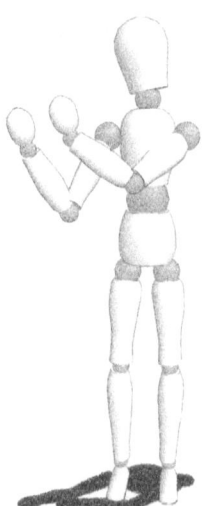

These instruments involve a clearly asymmetric posture with significant compromise of the shoulders, elbows, wrists, and fingers. In addition, the spinal column is at risk due to the twisting and inclined position that is often adopted.

Counterbalancing these strained postures and tensions by incorporating specific exercises is crucial for maintaining proper physical fitness.

## BEFORE PLAYING

**Essential**
(8 minutes 10 seconds total; 6 minutes without optional exercises)

| | | | |
|---|---|---|---|
| 1 | | Finger mobility 1<br>10 times (optional) | Page 29 |
| 12 | | Full arm rotations<br>10 times (optional) | Page 38 |
| 32 | | Yes with the neck<br>10 times (optional) | Page 57 |
| 33 | | Maybe with the neck<br>10 times (optional) | Page 58 |

# IN TUNE

| 34 | | No with the neck<br>10 times (optional) | Page 59 |
|---|---|---|---|
| 37 | | Side of the neck<br>20" + 20" | Page 61 |
| 38 | | Scapula levator<br>20" + 20" | Page 61 |
| 35 | | Back of the neck<br>20" + 20" (optional) | Page 59 |
| 36 | | Front of the neck<br>20" + 20" | Page 60 |
| 14 | | Fist out<br>20" + 20" | Page 40 |
| 16 | | Hand back<br>20" + 20" | Page 42 |
| 23 | | Latissimus dorsi<br>20" + 20" | Page 49 |

# CHAPTER FOUR EXERCISES BY INSTRUMENT

| | | | |
|---|---|---|---|
| 39 | | Interscapular<br>20" + 20" | Page 62 |
| 45 | | Lower back<br>20" + 20" | Page 68 |
| 24 | | Rear shoulder<br>20" + 20" | Page 50 |

## Complete
(14 minutes in total; 9 minutes 40 seconds without optional exercises)

| | | | |
|---|---|---|---|
| 1 | | Finger mobility 1<br>10 times | Page 29 |
| 2 | | Finger mobility 2<br>10 times (optional) | Page 30 |
| 19 | | Raising and lowering the shoulders<br>10 times (optional) | Page 46 |
| 12 | | Full arm rotations<br>10 times | Page 38 |

| | | | |
|---|---|---|---|
| 20 | | Twisting the chest and arms<br>10 times (optional) | Page 46 |
| 32 | | Yes with the neck<br>10 times (optional) | Page 57 |
| 33 | | Maybe with the neck<br>10 times (optional) | Page 58 |
| 34 | | No with the neck<br>10 times | Page 59 |
| 37 | | Side of the neck<br>20" + 20" | Page 61 |
| 38 | | Scapula levator<br>20" + 20" | Page 61 |
| 35 | | Back of the neck<br>20" + 20" (optional) | Page 59 |
| 36 | | Front of the neck<br>20" + 20" | Page 60 |

# CHAPTER FOUR

## EXERCISES BY INSTRUMENT

| | | | |
|---|---|---|---|
| 14 | | Fist out<br>20" + 20" | Page 40 |
| 16 | | Hand back<br>20" + 20" | Page 42 |
| 59 | | Vowels and consonants<br>30" | Page 79 |
| 60 | | One-sided face stretch<br>20" + 20" + 20" + 20" | Page 80 |
| 61 | | Two-sided face stretch<br>20" + 20" (optional) | Page 81 |
| 23 | | Latissimus dorsi<br>20" + 20" | Page 49 |
| 39 | | Interscapular<br>20" + 20" | Page 62 |
| 45 | | Lower back<br>20" + 20" | Page 68 |

**IN TUNE**

| 24 | 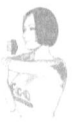 | Rear shoulder<br>20" + 20" | Page 50 |

# AFTER PLAYING

**Essential**
(6 minutes 40 seconds in total; 6 minutes without optional exercises)

| 37 | | Side of the neck<br>20" + 20" | Page 61 |
| 38 | | Scapula levator<br>20" + 20" | Page 61 |
| 35 | | Back of the neck<br>20" + 20" (optional) | Page 59 |
| 36 | | Front of the neck<br>20" + 20" | Page 60 |
| 15 | | Fist in<br>20" + 20" | Page 41 |
| 17 | | Hand down<br>20" + 20" | Page 42 |

**CHAPTER FOUR**  EXERCISES BY INSTRUMENT

| 23 | | Latissimus dorsi<br>20" + 20" | Page 49 |
| 39 | | Interscapular<br>20" + 20" | Page 62 |
| 45 | | Lower back<br>20" + 20" | Page 68 |
| 24 | | Rear shoulder<br>20" + 20" | Page 50 |

## Complete
(8 minutes 40 seconds total; 7 minutes 20 seconds without optional exercises)

| 37 | | Side of the neck<br>20" + 20" | Page 61 |
| 38 | | Scapula levator<br>20" + 20" | Page 61 |
| 35 | | Back of the neck<br>20" + 20" (optional) | Page 59 |

# IN TUNE

| | | | |
|---|---|---|---|
| 36 | | Front of the neck<br>20" + 20" | Page 60 |
| 15 | | Fist in<br>20" + 20" | Page 41 |
| 17 | | Hand down<br>20" + 20" | Page 42 |
| 60 | | One-sided face stretch<br>20" + 20" + 20" + 20" | Page 80 |
| 61 | | Two-sided face stretch<br>20" + 20" (optional) | Page 81 |
| 23 | | Latissimus dorsi<br>20" + 20" | Page 49 |
| 39 | | Interscapular<br>20" + 20" | Page 62 |
| 45 | | Lower back<br>20" + 20" | Page 68 |

**CHAPTER FOUR**                                              **EXERCISES BY INSTRUMENT**

| 24 | 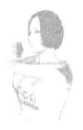 | Rear shoulder<br>20" + 20" | Page 50 |

# GROUP 5
# BOWED STRING, FRONT

The advantage of being able to rest the weight of the instrument is offset by significant stress on the left hand, asymmetric posture, *flexed elbows*, and a certain tendency to *close the shoulders*.

In order to avoid any possible problems, it is crucial to work these areas specifically.

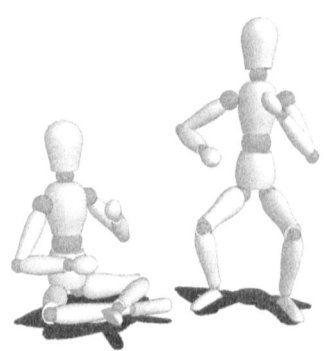

## BEFORE PLAYING

### Essential
(7 minutes 10 seconds in total; 5 minutes without optional exercises)

| | | | |
|---|---|---|---|
| 1 | | Finger mobility 1<br>10 times (optional) | Page 29 |
| 12 | | Full arm rotations<br>10 times (optional) | Page 38 |
| 32 | | Yes with the neck<br>10 times (optional) | Page 57 |
| 33 | | Maybe with the neck<br>10 times (optional) | Page 58 |

# CHAPTER FOUR — EXERCISES BY INSTRUMENT

| 34 | | No with the neck<br>10 times (optional) | Page 59 |
|---|---|---|---|
| 37 | | Side of the neck<br>20" + 20" | Page 61 |
| 38 | | Scapula levator<br>20" + 20" | Page 61 |
| 35 | | Back of the neck<br>20" + 20" (optional) | Page 59 |
| 36 | | Front of the neck<br>20" + 20" | Page 60 |
| 15 | | Fist in<br>20" + 20" | Page 41 |
| 17 | | Hand down<br>20" + 20" | Page 42 |
| 18 | | Hand inclined<br>20" + 20" | Page 43 |

**IN TUNE**

| 21 | | Chest<br>20" + 20" | Page 47 |
|---|---|---|---|
| 43 | | Back<br>20" | Page 66 |

**Complete**
(11 minutes 40 seconds in total; 8 minutes 30 seconds without optional exercises)

| 1 | | Finger mobility 1<br>10 times | Page 29 |
|---|---|---|---|
| 2 | | Finger mobility 2<br>10 times (optional) | Page 30 |
| 19 | | Raising and lowering the shoulders<br>10 times (optional) | Page 46 |
| 12 | | Full arm rotations<br>10 times | Page 38 |
| 20 | | Twisting the chest and arms<br>10 times (optional) | Page 46 |

# CHAPTER FOUR — EXERCISES BY INSTRUMENT

| 32 | Yes with the neck<br>10 times (optional) | Page 57 |
| 33 | Maybe with the neck<br>10 times (optional) | Page 58 |
| 34 | No with the neck<br>10 times | Page 59 |
| 37 | Side of the neck<br>20" + 20" | Page 61 |
| 38 | Scapula levator<br>20" + 20" | Page 61 |
| 35 | Back of the neck<br>20" + 20" | Page 59 |
| 36 | Front of the neck<br>20" + 20" (optional) | Page 60 |
| 15 | Fist in<br>20" + 20" | Page 41 |

# IN TUNE

| 17 | | Hand down<br>20" + 20" | Page 42 |
|---|---|---|---|
| 18 | | Hand inclined<br>20" + 20" | Page 43 |
| 21 | | Chest<br>20" + 20" | Page 47 |
| 43 | | Back<br>20" | Page 66 |
| 3 | | Hand muscles<br>20" + 20" + 20" + 20" | Page 31 |
| 4 | | Palm of the hand<br>20" | Page 31 |
| 44 | | Lateral abdominal muscles<br>20" + 20" | Page 67 |

# CHAPTER FOUR

EXERCISES BY INSTRUMENT

# AFTER PLAYING

## Essential
(5 minutes 40 seconds in total; 5 min without optional exercises)

| 37 | | Side of the neck<br>20" + 20" | Page 61 |
|---|---|---|---|
| 38 | | Scapula levator<br>20" + 20" | Page 61 |
| 35 | | Back of the neck<br>20" + 20" (optional) | Page 59 |
| 36 | | Front of the neck<br>20" + 20" | Page 60 |
| 14 | | Fist out<br>20" + 20" | Page 40 |
| 16 | | Hand back<br>20" + 20" | Page 42 |
| 18 | | Hand inclined<br>20" + 20" | Page 43 |

## IN TUNE

| 21 | | Chest<br>20" + 20" | Page 47 |
|---|---|---|---|
| 43 | | Back<br>20" | Page 66 |

**Complete**
(8 minutes in total; 6 minutes without optional exercises)

| 37 | | Side of the neck<br>20" + 20" | Page 61 |
|---|---|---|---|
| 38 | | Scapula levator<br>20" + 20" | Page 61 |
| 35 | | Back of the neck<br>20" + 20" (optional) | Page 59 |
| 36 | | Front of the neck<br>20" + 20" | Page 60 |
| 14 | | Fist out<br>20" + 20" | Page 40 |

# CHAPTER FOUR

**EXERCISES BY INSTRUMENT**

| | | | |
|---|---|---|---|
| 16 | | Hand back<br>20" + 20" | Page 42 |
| 18 | | Hand inclined<br>20" + 20" | Page 43 |
| 21 | | Chest<br>20" + 20" | Page 47 |
| 43 | | Back<br>20" | Page 66 |
| 3 | | Hand muscles<br>20" + 20" + 20" + 20" (optional) | Page 31 |
| 4 | | Palm of the hand<br>20" | Page 31 |
| 44 | | Lateral abdominal muscles<br>20" + 20" | Page 67 |

# GROUP 6
# LARGE BOWED STRING

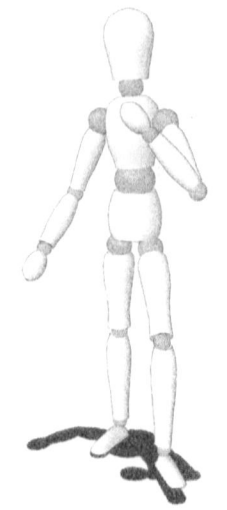

Even though the instrument can be played in a central position, the size tends to result in an asymmetric posture with the back generally tilted forward and to one side.

This program pays special attention to the most stressed zones, specifically the back but also the arms and hands, in order to maintain freedom from pain and reduced function.

## BEFORE PLAYING

**Essential**
(7 minutes 50 seconds in total; 5 minutes 40 seconds without optional exercises)

| 1 | | Finger mobility 1<br>10 times (optional) | Page 29 |
|---|---|---|---|
| 12 | | Full arm rotations<br>10 times (optional) | Page 38 |
| 32 | | Yes with the neck<br>10 times (optional) | Page 57 |
| 33 | | Maybe with the neck<br>10 times (optional) | Page 58 |

**CHAPTER FOUR**                                                  **EXERCISES BY INSTRUMENT**

| # | Exercise | Reference |
|---|---|---|
| 34 | No with the neck<br>10 times (optional) | Page 59 |
| 37 | Side of the neck<br>20" + 20" | Page 61 |
| 38 | Scapula levator<br>20" + 20" | Page 61 |
| 35 | Back of the neck<br>20" + 20" (optional) | Page 59 |
| 36 | Front of the neck<br>20" + 20" | Page 60 |
| 14 | Fist out<br>20" + 20" | Page 40 |
| 16 | Hand back<br>20" + 20" | Page 42 |
| 45 | Lower back<br>20" + 20" | Page 68 |

**IN TUNE**

| 43 | | Back 20" | Page 66 |
|---|---|---|---|
| 44 | | Lateral abdominal muscles 20" + 20" | Page 67 |
| 39 | | Interscapular 20" + 20" | Page 62 |

## Complete

(11 minutes 40 seconds in total; 8 minutes 20 seconds without optional exercises)

| 1 | | Finger mobility 1 10 times | Page 29 |
|---|---|---|---|
| 2 | | Finger mobility 2 10 times (optional) | Page 30 |
| 19 | | Raising and lowering the shoulders 10 times (optional) | Page 46 |
| 12 | | Full arm rotations 10 times | Page 38 |

# CHAPTER FOUR — EXERCISES BY INSTRUMENT

| 20 | Twisting the chest and arms<br>10 times (optional) | Page 46 |
| 32 | Yes with the neck<br>10 times (optional) | Page 57 |
| 33 | Maybe with the neck<br>10 times (optional) | Page 58 |
| 34 | No with the neck<br>10 times | Page 59 |
| 37 | Side of the neck<br>20" + 20" | Page 61 |
| 38 | Scapula levator<br>20" + 20" | Page 61 |
| 35 | Back of the neck<br>20" + 20" (optional) | Page 59 |
| 36 | Front of the neck<br>20" + 20" | Page 60 |

# IN TUNE

| 14 | Fist out<br>20" + 20" | Page 40 |
|---|---|---|
| 16 | Hand back<br>20" + 20" | Page 42 |
| 45 | Lower back<br>20" + 20" | Page 68 |
| 43 | Back<br>20" | Page 66 |
| 44 | Lateral abdominal muscles<br>20" + 20" | Page 67 |
| 39 | Interscapular<br>20" + 20" | Page 62 |
| 23 | Latissimus dorsi<br>20" + 20" | Page 49 |
| 21 | Chest<br>20" + 20" | Page 47 |

| | | | |
|---|---|---|---|
| 4 | 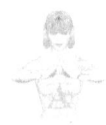 | Palm of the hand<br>20" | Page 31 |

# AFTER PLAYING

**Essential**
(6 minutes 20 seconds in total; 5 minutes 40 seconds without optional exercises)

| | | | |
|---|---|---|---|
| 37 | | Side of the neck<br>20" + 20" | Page 61 |
| 38 | | Scapula levator<br>20" + 20" | Page 61 |
| 35 | | Back of the neck<br>20" + 20" (optional) | Page 59 |
| 36 | | Front of the neck<br>20" + 20" | Page 60 |
| 15 | | Fist in<br>20" + 20" | Page 41 |
| 17 | | Hand down<br>20" + 20" | Page 42 |

| 45 | | Lower back  20" + 20" | Page 68 |
|---|---|---|---|
| 43 | | Back  20" | Page 66 |
| 44 | | Lateral abdominal muscles  20" + 20" | Page 67 |
| 39 | | Interscapular  20" + 20" | Page 62 |

## Complete
(8 minutes in total; 7 minutes 20 seconds without optional exercises)

| 37 | | Side of the neck  20" + 20" | Page 61 |
|---|---|---|---|
| 38 | | Scapula levator  20" + 20" | Page 61 |
| 35 | | Back of the neck  20" + 20" (optional) | Page 59 |

# CHAPTER FOUR                                    EXERCISES BY INSTRUMENT

| 36 | | Front of the neck<br>20" + 20" | Page 60 |
|----|---|---|---|
| 15 | | Fist in<br>20" + 20" | Page 41 |
| 17 | | Hand down<br>20" + 20" | Page 42 |
| 45 | | Lower back<br>20" + 20" | Page 68 |
| 43 | | Back<br>20" | Page 66 |
| 44 | | Lateral abdominal muscles<br>20" + 20" | Page 67 |
| 39 | | Interscapular<br>20" + 20" | Page 62 |
| 23 | | Latissimus dorsi<br>20" + 20" | Page 49 |

**IN TUNE**

| 21 | | Chest<br>20" + 20" | Page 47 |
|---|---|---|---|

| 4 | | Palm of the hand<br>20" | Page 31 |
|---|---|---|---|

CHAPTER FOUR                                    EXERCISES BY INSTRUMENT

# GROUP 7
# BOWED STRING, SHOULDER

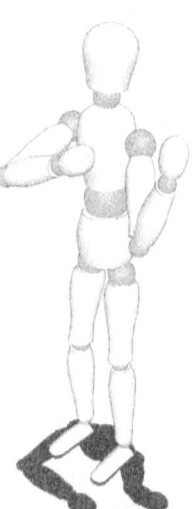

Bowed string instruments held in an asymmetric posture between the shoulder and the neck often create tension within the spinal column. In addition, the position and movement of the arms, especially the left, tend to strain the muscles of the forearm and the shoulder while compromising the elbow and wrist.

It is therefore essential to include exercises in this program aimed at counterbalancing the stresses generated in these areas.

## BEFORE PLAYING

**Essential**
(7 minutes 30 seconds in total; 5 minutes 20 seconds without optional exercises)

| | | | |
|---|---|---|---|
| 1 | | Finger mobility 1<br>10 times (optional) | Page 29 |
| 12 | | Full arm rotations<br>10 times (optional) | Page 38 |
| 32 | | Yes with the neck<br>10 times (optional) | Page 57 |
| 33 | | Maybe with the neck<br>10 times (optional) | Page 58 |

## IN TUNE

| 34 | | No with the neck<br>10 times (optional) | Page 59 |
|---|---|---|---|
| 37 | | Side of the neck<br>20" + 20" | Page 61 |
| 38 | | Scapula levator<br>20" + 20" | Page 61 |
| 35 | | Back of the neck<br>20" + 20" (optional) | Page 59 |
| 36 | | Front of the neck<br>20" + 20" | Page 60 |
| 14 | | Fist out<br>20" + 20" | Page 40 |
| 16 | | Hand back<br>20" + 20" | Page 42 |
| 11 | | Ping-pong balls<br>3' | Page 37 |

| CHAPTER FOUR | | | EXERCISES BY INSTRUMENT | |
|---|---|---|---|---|
| 24 | 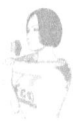 | Rear shoulder<br>20" + 20" | | Page 50 |
| 44 | 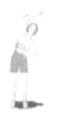 | Lateral abdominal muscles<br>20" + 20" | | Page 67 |

## Complete
(12 minutes 20 seconds; 7 minutes 50 seconds without optional exercises)

| 1 | | Finger mobility 1<br>10 times | | Page 29 |
|---|---|---|---|---|
| 2 | | Finger mobility 2<br>10 times (optional) | | Page 30 |
| 19 | | Raising and lowering shoulders<br>10 times (optional) | | Page 46 |
| 12 | | Full arm rotations<br>10 times | | Page 38 |
| 20 | | Twisting the chest and arms<br>10 times (optional) | | Page 46 |

**IN TUNE**

| | | | |
|---|---|---|---|
| 32 | | Yes with the neck<br>10 times (optional) | Page 57 |
| 33 | | Maybe with the neck<br>10 times (optional) | Page 58 |
| 34 | | No with the neck<br>10 times | Page 59 |
| 37 | | Side of the neck<br>20" + 20" | Page 61 |
| 38 | | Scapula levator<br>20" + 20" | Page 61 |
| 35 | | Back of the neck<br>20" + 20" (optional) | Page 59 |
| 36 | | Front of the neck<br>20" + 20" | Page 60 |
| 14 | | Fist out<br>20" + 20" | Page 40 |

**CHAPTER FOUR**              **EXERCISES BY INSTRUMENT**

| 16 | Hand back<br>20" + 20" | Page 42 |
|---|---|---|
| 21 | Chest<br>20" + 20" | Page 47 |
| 24 | Rear shoulder<br>20" + 20" | Page 50 |
| 44 | Lateral abdominal muscles<br>20" + 20" | Page 67 |
| 39 | Interscapular<br>20" + 20" | Page 62 |
| 3 | Hand muscles<br>20" + 20" + 20" + 20" (optional) | Page 31 |
| 4 | Palm of the hand<br>20" | Page 31 |
| 43 | Back<br>20" | Page 66 |

IN TUNE

# AFTER PLAYING

**Essential**
(6 minutes in total; 5 minutes 20 seconds without optional exercises)

| 37 | Side of the neck<br>20" + 20" | Page 61 |
|---|---|---|
| 38 | Scapula levator<br>20" + 20" | Page 61 |
| 35 | Back of the neck<br>20" + 20" (optional) | Page 59 |
| 36 | Front of the neck<br>20" + 20" | Page 60 |
| 15 | Fist in<br>20" + 20" | Page 41 |
| 17 | Hand down<br>20" + 20" | Page 42 |
| 21 | Chest<br>20" + 20" | Page 47 |

# CHAPTER FOUR                                    EXERCISES BY INSTRUMENT

| | | | |
|---|---|---|---|
| 24 | | Rear shoulder<br>20" + 20" | Page 50 |
| 44 | | Lateral abdominal muscles<br>20" + 20" | Page 67 |

**Complete**
(8 minutes 40 seconds in total; 6 minutes 40 seconds without optional exercises)

| | | | |
|---|---|---|---|
| 37 | | Side of the neck<br>20" + 20" | Page 61 |
| 38 | | Scapula levator<br>20" + 20" | Page 61 |
| 35 | | Back of the neck<br>20" + 20" (optional) | Page 59 |
| 36 | | Front of the neck<br>20" + 20" | Page 60 |
| 15 | | Fist in<br>20" + 20" | Page 41 |

# IN TUNE

| 17 | | Hand down<br>20" + 20" | Page 42 |
|---|---|---|---|
| 21 | | Chest<br>20" + 20" | Page 47 |
| 24 | | Rear shoulder<br>20" + 20" | Page 50 |
| 44 | | Lateral abdominal muscles<br>20" + 20" | Page 67 |
| 39 | | Interscapular<br>20" + 20" | Page 62 |
| 3 | | Hand muscles<br>20" + 20" + 20" + 20" (optional) | Page 31 |
| 4 | | Palm of the hand<br>20" | Page 31 |
| 43 | | Back<br>20" | Page 66 |

| CHAPTER FOUR | EXERCISES BY INSTRUMENT |

# GROUP 8
# PLUCKED STRING

Even though the posture is a little more symmetrical than other instruments, it still places a certain amount of stress on the back. The technical demands and the strained positions that are momentarily adopted when playing tend to overstress some joints and muscles.

All of this makes it crucial to incorporate a program to counterbalance these stresses to prevent any future problems.

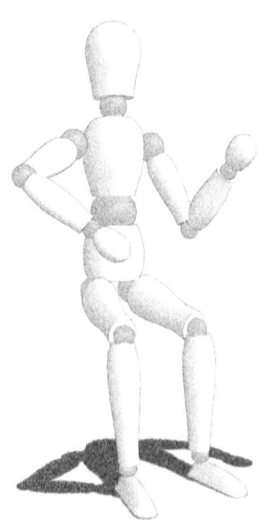

## BEFORE PLAYING

**Essential**
(8 minutes 30 seconds in total; 5 minutes 40 seconds without optional exercises)

| | | | |
|---|---|---|---|
| 1 | | Finger mobility 1<br>10 times (optional) | Page 29 |
| 12 | | Full arm rotations<br>10 times (optional) | Page 38 |
| 32 | | Yes with the neck<br>10 times (optional) | Page 57 |
| 33 | | Maybe with the neck<br>10 times (optional) | Page 58 |

## IN TUNE

| 34 | No with the neck<br>10 times (optional) | Page 59 |
| --- | --- | --- |
| 37 | Side of the neck<br>20" + 20" | Page 61 |
| 38 | Scapula levator<br>20" + 20" | Page 61 |
| 35 | Back of the neck<br>20" + 20" (optional) | Page 59 |
| 36 | Front of the neck<br>20" + 20" | Page 60 |
| 15 | Fist in<br>20" + 20" | Page 41 |
| 17 | Hand down<br>20" + 20" | Page 42 |
| 39 | Interscapular<br>20" + 20" | Page 62 |

# CHAPTER FOUR

**EXERCISES BY INSTRUMENT**

| 23 | | Latissimus dorsi<br>20" + 20" | Page 49 |
|---|---|---|---|
| 43 | | Back<br>20" | Page 66 |
| 5 | | Thumb down<br>20" + 20" (optional) | Page 32 |
| 6 | | Thumb back<br>20" + 20" | Page 33 |

## Complete

(13 minutes 40 seconds in total; 9 minutes 10 seconds without optional exercises)

| 1 | | Finger mobility 1<br>10 times | Page 29 |
|---|---|---|---|
| 2 | | Finger mobility 2<br>10 times (optional) | Page 30 |
| 19 | | Raising and lowering the shoulders<br>10 times (optional) | Page 46 |

159

# IN TUNE

| 12 | | Full arm rotations<br>10 times | Page 38 |
|---|---|---|---|
| 20 | | Twisting the chest and arms<br>10 times (optional) | Page 46 |
| 32 | | Yes with the neck<br>10 times (optional) | Page 57 |
| 33 | | Maybe with the neck<br>10 times (optional) | Page 58 |
| 34 | | No with the neck<br>10 times | Page 59 |
| 37 | | Side of the neck<br>20" + 20" | Page 61 |
| 38 | | Scapula levator<br>20" + 20" | Page 61 |
| 35 | | Back of the neck<br>20" + 20" (optional) | Page 59 |

# CHAPTER FOUR

**EXERCISES BY INSTRUMENT**

| | | | |
|---|---|---|---|
| 36 | | Front of the neck<br>20" + 20" | Page 60 |
| 15 | | Fist in<br>20" + 20" | Page 41 |
| 17 | | Hand down<br>20" + 20" | Page 42 |
| 39 | | Interscapular<br>20" + 20" | Page 62 |
| 23 | | Latissimus dorsi<br>20" + 20" | Page 49 |
| 43 | | Back<br>20" | Page 66 |
| 5 | | Thumb down<br>20" + 20" | Page 32 |
| 6 | | Thumb back<br>20" + 20" | Page 33 |

# IN TUNE

| 18 | Hand inclined<br>20" + 20" | Page 43 |
| 22 | Posterior arm muscles<br>20" + 20" | Page 48 |
| 4 | Palm of the hand<br>20" | Page 31 |
| 3 | Hand muscles<br>20" + 20" + 20" + 20" (optional) | Page 31 |

# AFTER PLAYING

**Essential**
(7 minutes in total; 5 minutes 40 seconds without optional exercises)

| 37 | Side of the neck<br>20" + 20" | Page 61 |
| 38 | Scapula levator<br>20" + 20" | Page 61 |
| 35 | Back of the neck<br>20" + 20" (optional) | Page 59 |

# CHAPTER FOUR

**EXERCISES BY INSTRUMENT**

| | | | |
|---|---|---|---|
| 36 | | Front of the neck<br>20" + 20" | Page 60 |
| 14 | | Fist out<br>20" + 20" | Page 40 |
| 16 | | Hand back<br>20" + 20" | Page 42 |
| 39 | | Interscapular<br>20" + 20" | Page 62 |
| 23 | | Latissimus dorsi<br>20" + 20" | Page 49 |
| 43 | | Back<br>20" | Page 66 |
| 5 | | Thumb down<br>20" + 20" | Page 32 |
| 6 | | Thumb back<br>20" + 20" | Page 33 |

# IN TUNE

**Complete**
(10 minutes in total; 8 minutes without optional exercises)

| 37 | | Side of the neck<br>20" + 20" | Page 61 |
|---|---|---|---|
| 38 | | Scapula levator<br>20" + 20" | Page 61 |
| 35 | | Back of the neck<br>20" + 20" (optional) | Page 59 |
| 36 | | Front of the neck<br>20" + 20" | Page 60 |
| 14 | | Fist out<br>20" + 20" | Page 40 |
| 16 | | Hand back<br>20" + 20" | Page 42 |
| 39 | | Interscapular<br>20" + 20" | Page 60 |

# CHAPTER FOUR

EXERCISES BY INSTRUMENT

| 23 | Latissimus dorsi<br>20" + 20" | Page 49 |
|---|---|---|
| 43 | Back<br>20" | Page 66 |
| 5 | Thumb down<br>20" + 20" | Page 32 |
| 6 | Thumb back<br>20" + 20" | Page 33 |
| 18 | Hand inclined<br>20" + 20" | Page 43 |
| 22 | Posterior arm muscles<br>20" + 20" | Page 48 |
| 4 | Palm of the hand<br>20" | Page 31 |
| 3 | Hand muscles<br>20" + 20" + 20" + 20" (optional) | Page 31 |

IN TUNE

# GROUP 9
# PLUCKED STRING, HARP

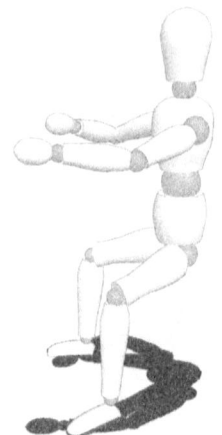

Having to play an instrument with the hands generally far away from the body, elbows raised, and specific movement of the feet often generates tension and overstresses the arms, shoulders, back, and hands. These musicians also tend to *close the shoulders,* sustaining them in a forward position that causes *dorsal hunching* and loss of the proper lumbar curve.

Incorporating exercises in this program that counterbalance these stresses are essential for maintaining a good quality of life.

## BEFORE PLAYING

**Essential**
(8 minutes 10 seconds in total; 5 minutes 20 seconds without optional exercises)

| | | | |
|---|---|---|---|
| 1 | | Finger mobility 1<br>10 times (optional) | Page 29 |
| 12 | | Full arm rotations<br>10 times (optional) | Page 38 |
| 32 | | Yes with the neck<br>10 times (optional) | Page 57 |
| 33 | | Maybe with the neck<br>10 times (optional) | Page 58 |

**CHAPTER FOUR**            **EXERCISES BY INSTRUMENT**

| | | | |
|---|---|---|---|
| 34 | | No with the neck<br>10 times (optional) | Page 59 |
| 37 | | Side of the neck<br>20" + 20" | Page 61 |
| 38 | | Scapula levator<br>20" + 20" | Page 61 |
| 35 | | Back of the neck<br>20" + 20" (optional) | Page 59 |
| 36 | | Front of the neck<br>20" + 20" | Page 60 |
| 14 | | Fist out<br>20" + 20" | Page 40 |
| 16 | | Hand back<br>20" + 20" | Page 42 |
| 21 | | Chest<br>20" + 20" | Page 47 |

# IN TUNE

| 22 | | Posterior arm muscles<br>20" + 20" | Page 48 |
|---|---|---|---|
| 23 | | Latissimus dorsi<br>20" + 20" | Page 49 |
| 52 | | Leg back 1<br>20" + 20" (optional) | Page 73 |

**Complete**
(11 minutes 40 seconds in total; 8 minutes 30 seconds without optional exercises)

| 1 | | Finger mobility 1<br>10 times (optional) | Page 29 |
|---|---|---|---|
| 2 | | Finger mobility 2<br>10 times (optional) | Page 30 |
| 19 | | Raising and lowering the shoulders<br>10 times (optional) | Page 46 |
| 12 | | Full arm rotations<br>10 times | Page 38 |

| **CHAPTER FOUR** | | | **EXERCISES BY INSTRUMENT** |
|---|---|---|---|
| 20 | | Twisting the chest and arms<br>10 times (optional) | Page 46 |
| 32 | | Yes with the neck<br>10 times (optional) | Page 57 |
| 33 | | Maybe with the neck<br>10 times (optional) | Page 58 |
| 34 | | No with the neck<br>10 times | Page 59 |
| 37 | | Side of the neck<br>20" + 20" | Page 61 |
| 38 | | Scapula levator<br>20" + 20" | Page 61 |
| 35 | | Back of the neck<br>20" + 20" (optional) | Page 59 |
| 36 | | Front of the neck<br>20" + 20" | Page 60 |

**IN TUNE**

| 14 | | Fist out 20" + 20" | Page 40 |
|---|---|---|---|
| 16 | | Hand back 20" + 20" | Page 42 |
| 21 | | Chest 20" + 20" | Page 47 |
| 22 | | Posterior arm muscles 20" + 20" | Page 48 |
| 23 | | Latissimus dorsi 20" + 20" | Page 49 |
| 52 | | Leg back 1 20" + 20" (optional) | Page 73 |
| 4 | | Palm of the hand 20" | Page 31 |
| 43 | | Back 20" | Page 66 |

| 44 | 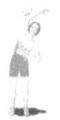 | Lateral abdominal muscles<br>20" + 20" | Page 67 |

## AFTER PLAYING

**Essential**
(6 minutes 40 seconds in total; 5 minutes 20 seconds without optional exercises)

| 37 | | Side of the neck<br>20" + 20" | Page 61 |
| 38 | | Scapula levator<br>20" + 20" | Page 61 |
| 35 | | Back of the neck<br>20" + 20" (optional) | Page 59 |
| 36 | | Front of the neck<br>20" + 20" | Page 60 |
| 15 | | Fist in<br>20" + 20" | Page 41 |
| 17 | | Hand down<br>20" + 20" | Page 42 |

**IN TUNE**

| 21 | | Chest<br>20" + 20" | Page 47 |
|---|---|---|---|
| 22 | | Posterior arm muscles<br>20" + 20" | Page 48 |
| 23 | | Latissimus dorsi<br>20" + 20" | Page 49 |
| 52 | | Leg back 1<br>20" + 20" (optional) | Page 73 |

**Complete**
(8 minutes in total; 7 minutes 20 seconds without optional exercises)

| 37 | | Side of the neck<br>20" + 20" | Page 61 |
|---|---|---|---|
| 38 | | Scapula levator<br>20" + 20" | Page 61 |
| 35 | | Back of the neck<br>20" + 20" (optional) | Page 59 |

| CHAPTER FOUR | | | EXERCISES BY INSTRUMENT |
|---|---|---|---|
| 36 | | Front of the neck<br>20" + 20" | Page 60 |
| 15 | | Fist in<br>20" + 20" | Page 41 |
| 17 | | Hand down<br>20" + 20" | Page 42 |
| 21 | | Chest<br>20" + 20" | Page 47 |
| 22 | | Posterior arm muscles<br>20" + 20" | Page 48 |
| 23 | | Latissimus dorsi<br>20" + 20" | Page 49 |
| 52 | | Leg back 1<br>20" + 20" | Page 73 |
| 4 | | Palm of the hand<br>20" | Page 31 |

| 43 | 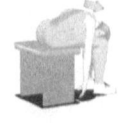 | Back<br>20" | Page 66 |
| 44 |  | Lateral abdominal muscles<br>20" + 20" | Page 67 |

CHAPTER FOUR                                           EXERCISES BY INSTRUMENT

# GROUP 10
# PERCUSSION

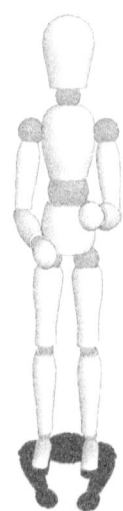

Even though some percussion instruments allow a relatively symmetrical and balanced posture, the energy and the repeated impacts, however small they may be, end up overstressing the spinal column and the upper extremities.

It is important to counterbalance these stresses with exercises designed specifically for these areas.

## BEFORE PLAYING

### Essential
(6 minutes 50 seconds in total; 4 minutes 40 seconds without optional exercises)

| | | | |
|---|---|---|---|
| 1 | | Finger mobility 1<br>10 times (optional) | Page 29 |
| 12 | | Full arm rotations<br>10 times (optional) | Page 38 |
| 32 | | Yes with the neck<br>10 times (optional) | Page 57 |
| 33 | | Maybe with the neck<br>10 times (optional) | Page 58 |

| | | | |
|---|---|---|---|
| 34 | | No with the neck<br>10 times (optional) | Page 59 |
| 37 | | Side of the neck<br>20" + 20" | Page 61 |
| 38 | | Scapula levator<br>20" + 20" | Page 61 |
| 35 | | Back of the neck<br>20" + 20" (optional) | Page 59 |
| 36 | | Front of the neck<br>20" + 20" | Page 60 |
| 14 | | Fist out<br>20" + 20" | Page 40 |
| 16 | | Hand back<br>20" + 20" | Page 42 |
| 43 | | Back<br>20" | Page 66 |

| CHAPTER FOUR | | | EXERCISES BY INSTRUMENT |
|---|---|---|---|

| 45 | | Lower back<br>20" + 20" | Page 68 |
|---|---|---|---|
| 4 | | Palm of the hand<br>20" | Page 31 |

## Complete
(12 minutes 20 seconds in total; 7 minutes 50 seconds without optional exercises)

| 1 | | Finger mobility 1<br>10 times | Page 29 |
|---|---|---|---|
| 2 | | Finger mobility 2<br>10 times (optional) | Page 30 |
| 19 | | Raising and lowering the shoulders<br>10 times (optional) | Page 46 |
| 12 | | Full arm rotations<br>10 times | Page 38 |
| 20 | | Twisting the chest and arms<br>10 times (optional) | Page 46 |

**IN TUNE**

| | | | |
|---|---|---|---|
| 32 | | Yes with the neck<br>10 times (optional) | Page 57 |
| 33 | | Maybe with the neck<br>10 times (optional) | Page 58 |
| 34 | | No with the neck<br>10 times | Page 59 |
| 37 | | Side of the neck<br>20" + 20" | Page 51 |
| 38 | | Scapula levator<br>20" + 20" | Page 61 |
| 35 | | Back of the neck<br>20" + 20" (optional) | Page 59 |
| 36 | | Front of the neck<br>20" + 20" | Page 60 |
| 14 | | Fist out<br>20" + 20" | Page 40 |

**CHAPTER FOUR**            EXERCISES BY INSTRUMENT

| # | | Exercise | Page |
|---|---|---|---|
| 16 | | Hand back<br>20" + 20" | Page 42 |
| 43 | | Back<br>20" | Page 66 |
| 45 | | Lower back<br>20" + 20" | Page 68 |
| 4 | | Palm of the hand<br>20" | Page 31 |
| 3 | | Hand muscles<br>20" + 20" + 20" + 20" (optional) | Page 31 |
| 44 | | Lateral abdominal muscles<br>20" + 20" | Page 67 |
| 22 | | Posterior arm muscles<br>20" + 20" | Page 48 |
| 23 | | Latissimus dorsi<br>20" + 20" | Page 49 |

# IN TUNE

# AFTER PLAYING

**Essential**
(5 minutes 20 seconds in total; 4 minutes 40 seconds without optional exercises)

| 37 | Side of the neck<br>20" + 20" | Page 61 |
|---|---|---|
| 38 | Scapula levator<br>20" + 20" | Page 61 |
| 35 | Back of the neck<br>20" + 20" (optional) | Page 59 |
| 36 | Front of the neck<br>20" + 20" | Page 60 |
| 15 | Fist in<br>20" + 20" | Page 41 |
| 17 | Hand down<br>20" + 20" | Page 42 |
| 43 | Back<br>20" | Page 66 |

# CHAPTER FOUR — EXERCISES BY INSTRUMENT

| 45 | Lower back  20" + 20" | Page 68 |

| 4 | Palm of the hand  20" | Page 31 |

## Complete
(8 minutes 40 seconds in total; 6 minutes 40 seconds without optional exercises)

| 37 | Side of the neck  20" + 20" | Page 61 |

| 38 | Scapula levator  20" + 20" | Page 61 |

| 35 | Back of the neck  20" + 20" (optional) | Page 59 |

| 36 | Front of the neck  20" + 20" | Page 60 |

| 15 | Fist in  20" + 20" | Page 41 |

| | | | | |
|---|---|---|---|---|
| 17 | | Hand down<br>20" + 20" | | Page 42 |
| 43 | | Back<br>20" | | Page 66 |
| 45 | | Lower back<br>20" + 20" | | Page 68 |
| 4 | | Palm of the hand<br>20" | | Page 31 |
| 3 | | Hand muscles<br>20" + 20" + 20" + 20" (optional) | | Page 31 |
| 44 | | Lateral abdominal muscles<br>20" + 20" | | Page 67 |
| 22 | | Posterior arm muscle<br>20" + 20" | | Page 48 |
| 23 | | Latissimus dorsi<br>20" + 20" | | Page 49 |

# CHAPTER FOUR        EXERCISES BY INSTRUMENT

# GROUP 11
# PERCUSSION, DRUM SET

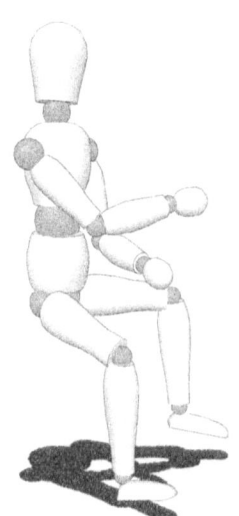

The simultaneous work of the arms and legs at different levels and distances makes it difficult to maintain a good base of support. This results in significant stress to the spinal column.

In order to avoid any possible problems, it is crucial to regularly exercise these areas, along with the arms and shoulders.

## BEFORE PLAYING

### Essential
(8 minutes 50 seconds in total; 6 minutes 40 seconds without optional exercises)

| | | | |
|---|---|---|---|
| 1 | | Finger mobility 1<br>10 times (optional) | Page 29 |
| 12 | | Full arm rotations<br>10 times (optional) | Page 38 |
| 32 | | Yes with the neck<br>10 times (optional) | Page 57 |
| 33 | | Maybe with the neck<br>10 times (optional) | Page 58 |

**IN TUNE**

| | | | |
|---|---|---|---|
| 34 | | No with the neck<br>10 times (optional) | Page 59 |
| 37 | | Side of the neck<br>20" + 20" | Page 61 |
| 38 | | Scapula levator<br>20" + 20" | Page 61 |
| 35 | | Back of the neck<br>20" + 20" (optional) | Page 59 |
| 36 | | Front of the neck<br>20" + 20" | Page 60 |
| 15 | | Fist in<br>20" + 20" | Page 41 |
| 17 | | Hand down<br>20" + 20" | Page 42 |
| 13 | | Wrist down<br>20" + 20" | Page 39 |

| CHAPTER FOUR | | | EXERCISES BY INSTRUMENT |
|---|---|---|---|

| 18 | | Hand inclined<br>20" + 20" | Page 43 |
|---|---|---|---|
| 45 | | Lower back<br>20" + 20" | Page 68 |
| 23 | | Latissimus dorsi<br>20" + 20" | Page 49 |
| 52 | | Leg back 1<br>20" + 20" | Page 73 |

**Complete**
(12 minutes 40 seconds in total; 9 minutes 30 seconds without optional exercises)

| 1 | | Finger mobility 1<br>10 times | Page 29 |
|---|---|---|---|
| 2 | | Finger mobility 2<br>10 times (optional) | Page 30 |
| 19 | | Raising and lowering the shoulders<br>10 times (optional) | Page 46 |

# IN TUNE

| 12 | Full arm rotations 10 times | Page 38 |
| 20 | Twisting the chest and arms 10 times (optional) | Page 46 |
| 32 | Yes with the neck 10 times (optional) | Page 57 |
| 33 | Maybe with the neck 10 times (optional) | Page 58 |
| 34 | No with the neck 10 times | Page 59 |
| 37 | Side of the neck 20" + 20" | Page 61 |
| 38 | Scapula levator 20" + 20" | Page 61 |
| 35 | Back of the neck 20" + 20" (optional) | Page 59 |

# CHAPTER FOUR

## EXERCISES BY INSTRUMENT

| 36 | | Front of the neck<br>20" + 20" | Page 60 |
|---|---|---|---|
| 15 | | Fist in<br>20" + 20" | Page 41 |
| 17 | | Hand down<br>20" + 20" | Page 42 |
| 13 | | Wrist down<br>20" + 20" | Page 39 |
| 18 | | Hand inclined<br>20" + 20" | Page 43 |
| 45 | | Lower back<br>20" + 20" | Page 68 |
| 23 | | Latissimus dorsi<br>20" + 20" | Page 49 |
| 52 | | Leg back 1<br>20" + 20" | Page 73 |

# IN TUNE

| 44 | | Lateral abdominal muscles<br>20" + 20" | Page 67 |
|---|---|---|---|
| 22 | | Posterior arm muscles<br>20" + 20" | Page 48 |
| 43 | | Back<br>20" | Page 66 |

## AFTER PLAYING

**Essential**
(7 minutes 20 seconds in total; 6 minutes 40 seconds without optional exercises)

| 37 | | Side of the neck<br>20" + 20" | Page 61 |
|---|---|---|---|
| 38 | | Scapula levator<br>20" + 20" | Page 61 |
| 35 | | Back of the neck<br>20" + 20" (optional) | Page 59 |
| 36 | | Front of the neck<br>20" + 20" | Page 60 |

# CHAPTER FOUR — EXERCISES BY INSTRUMENT

| 14 | Fist out<br>20" + 20" | Page 40 |
|---|---|---|
| 16 | Hand back<br>20" + 20" | Page 42 |
| 13 | Wrist down<br>20" + 20" | Page 39 |
| 18 | Hand inclined<br>20" + 20" | Page 43 |
| 45 | Lower back<br>20" + 20" | Page 68 |
| 23 | Latissimus dorsi<br>20" + 20" | Page 49 |
| 52 | Leg back 1<br>20" + 20" | Page 73 |

**IN TUNE**

**Complete**

(13 minutes in total; 12 minutes 20 seconds without optional exercises)

| 37 | | Side of the neck<br>20" + 20" | Page 61 |
|---|---|---|---|
| 38 | | Scapula levator<br>20" + 20" | Page 61 |
| 35 | | Back of the neck<br>20" + 20" (optional) | Page 59 |
| 36 | | Front of the neck<br>20" + 20" | Page 60 |
| 14 | | Fist out<br>20" + 20" | Page 40 |
| 16 | | Hand back<br>20" + 20" | Page 42 |
| 13 | | Wrist down<br>20" + 20" | Page 39 |

| CHAPTER FOUR | | | EXERCISES BY INSTRUMENT |
|---|---|---|---|
| 18 | | Hand inclined<br>20" + 20" | Page 43 |
| 45 | | Lower back<br>20" + 20" | Page 68 |
| 23 | | Latissimus dorsi<br>20" + 20" | Page 49 |
| 52 | | Leg back I<br>20" + 20" | Page 73 |
| 44 | | Lateral abdominal muscles<br>20" + 20" | Page 67 |
| 22 | | Posterior arm muscles<br>20" + 20" | Page 48 |
| 43 | | Back<br>20" | Page 66 |

# GROUP 12
# KEYBOARD

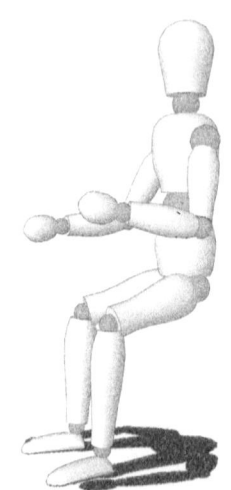

When playing keyboard instruments, more attention is often given to the fingers than the other areas of the body. It is a common misunderstanding that these other areas do not suffer as much because they are worked in symmetrical and ergonomic postures.

The back, along with the hands and forearms, should be kept in shape as it is an area where tensions and stresses generally accumulate.

## BEFORE PLAYING

**Essential**
(6 minutes 50 seconds in total; 4 minutes 40 seconds without optional exercises)

| 1 | | Finger mobility 1<br>10 times (optional) | Page 29 |
|---|---|---|---|
| 12 | | Full arm rotations<br>10 times (optional) | Page 38 |
| 32 | | Yes with the neck<br>10 times (optional) | Page 57 |
| 33 | | Maybe with the neck<br>10 times (optional) | Page 58 |

# CHAPTER FOUR

**EXERCISES BY INSTRUMENT**

| 34 | | No with the neck<br>10 times (optional) | Page 59 |
|---|---|---|---|
| 37 | | Side of the neck<br>20" + 20" | Page 61 |
| 38 | | Scapula levator<br>20" + 20" | Page 61 |
| 35 | | Back of the neck<br>20" + 20" (optional) | Page 59 |
| 36 | | Front of the neck<br>20" + 20" | Page 60 |
| 15 | | Fist in<br>20" + 20" | Page 41 |
| 17 | | Hand down<br>20" + 20" | Page 42 |
| 18 | | Hand inclined<br>20" + 20" | Page 43 |

# IN TUNE

| 43 | | Back<br>20" | Page 66 |
|---|---|---|---|
| 4 | | Palm of the hand<br>20" | Page 31 |

## Complete
(11 minutes 40 seconds in total; 7 minutes 10 seconds without optional exercises)

| 1 | | Finger mobility 1<br>10 times | Page 29 |
|---|---|---|---|
| 2 | | Finger mobility 2<br>10 times (optional) | Page 30 |
| 19 | | Raising and lowering the shoulders<br>10 times (optional) | Page 46 |
| 12 | | Full arm rotations<br>10 times | Page 38 |
| 20 | | Twisting the chest and arms<br>10 times (optional) | Page 46 |

**CHAPTER FOUR**　　　　　　　　　　　　　　　　　　　　**EXERCISES BY INSTRUMENT**

| | | | |
|---|---|---|---|
| 32 | | Yes with the neck<br>10 times (optional) | Page 57 |
| 33 | | Maybe with the neck<br>10 times (optional) | Page 58 |
| 34 | | No with the neck<br>10 times | Page 59 |
| 37 | | Side of the neck<br>20" + 20" | Page 61 |
| 38 | | Scapula levator<br>20" + 20" | Page 61 |
| 35 | | Back of the neck<br>20" + 20" (optional) | Page 59 |
| 36 | | Front of the neck<br>20" + 20" | Page 60 |
| 15 | | Fist in<br>20" + 20" | Page 41 |

# IN TUNE

| 17 | | Hand down<br>20" + 20" | Page 42 |
| --- | --- | --- | --- |
| 18 | | Hand inclined<br>20" + 20" | Page 43 |
| 43 | | Back<br>20" | Page 66 |
| 4 | | Palm of the hand<br>20" | Page 31 |
| 13 | | Wrist down<br>20" + 20" | Page 39 |
| 23 | | Latissimus dorsi<br>20" + 20" | Page 49 |
| 3 | | Hand muscles<br>20" + 20" + 20" + 20" (optional) | Page 31 |

**CHAPTER FOUR**  EXERCISES BY INSTRUMENT

# AFTER PLAYING

**Essential**
(5 minutes 20 seconds in total; 4 minutes 40 seconds without optional exercises)

| 37 | | Side of the neck<br>20" + 20" | Page 61 |
|---|---|---|---|
| 38 | | Scapula levator<br>20" + 20" | Page 61 |
| 35 | | Back of the neck<br>20" + 20" (optional) | Page 59 |
| 36 | | Front of the neck<br>20" + 20" | Page 60 |
| 14 | | Fist out<br>20" + 20" | Page 40 |
| 16 | | Hand back<br>20" + 20" | Page 42 |
| 18 | | Hand inclined<br>20" + 20" | Page 43 |

# IN TUNE

| 43 | | Back<br>20" | Page 66 |
|---|---|---|---|
| 4 | | Palm of the hand<br>20" | Page 31 |

## Complete
(8 minutes in total; 6 minutes without optional exercises)

| 37 | | Side of the neck<br>20" + 20" | Page 61 |
|---|---|---|---|
| 38 | | Scapula levator<br>20" + 20" | Page 61 |
| 35 | | Back of the neck<br>20" + 20" (optional) | Page 59 |
| 36 | | Front of the neck<br>20" + 20" | Page 60 |
| 14 | | Fist out<br>20" + 20" | Page 40 |

# CHAPTER FOUR

EXERCISES BY INSTRUMENT

| | | | |
|---|---|---|---|
| 16 | | Hand back<br>20" + 20" | Page 42 |
| 18 | | Hand inclined<br>20" + 20" | Page 43 |
| 43 | | Back<br>20" | Page 66 |
| 4 | | Palm of the hand<br>20" | Page 31 |
| 13 | | Wrist down<br>20" + 20" | Page 39 |
| 23 | | Latissimus dorsi<br>20" + 20" | Page 49 |
| 3 | | Hand muscles<br>20" + 20" + 20" + 20" (optional) | Page 31 |

# IN TUNE

# GROUP 13
# KEYBOARD
# WITH HANDS AND FEET

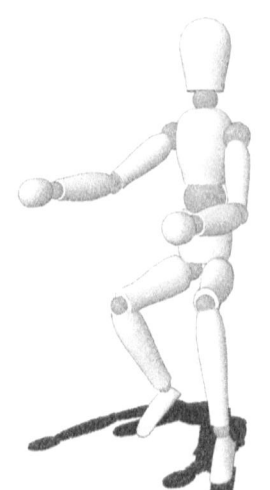

These instruments levy a significant demand on the entire spinal column due to the simultaneous work of the arms and legs, especially when considering that the feet lack proper support and the hands work at different heights and distances.

It is crucial to incorporate specific exercises that counterbalance the stresses to these areas.

## BEFORE PLAYING

**Essential**
(7 minutes 50 seconds in total; 5 minutes 40 seconds without optional exercises)

| 1 | | Finger mobility 1<br>10 times (optional) | Page 29 |
|---|---|---|---|
| 12 | | Full arm rotations<br>10 times (optional) | Page 38 |
| 32 | | Yes with the neck<br>10 times (optional) | Page 57 |
| 33 | | Maybe with the neck<br>10 times (optional) | Page 58 |

**CHAPTER FOUR**  EXERCISES BY INSTRUMENT

| 34 | | No with the neck<br>10 times (optional) | Page 59 |
| 37 | | Side of the neck<br>20" + 20" | Page 61 |
| 38 | | Scapula levator<br>20" + 20" | Page 61 |
| 35 | | Back of the neck<br>20" + 20" (optional) | Page 59 |
| 36 | | Front of the neck<br>20" + 20" | Page 60 |
| 14 | | Fist out<br>20" + 20" | Page 40 |
| 16 | | Hand back<br>20" + 20" | Page 42 |
| 21 | | Chest<br>20" + 20" | Page 47 |

## IN TUNE

| 45 | | Lower back<br>20" + 20" | Page 68 |
|---|---|---|---|

| 43 | | Back<br>20" | Page 66 |
|---|---|---|---|

| 52 | | Leg back 1<br>20" + 20" | Page 73 |
|---|---|---|---|

### Complete
(11 minutes 40 seconds in total; 8 minutes 20 seconds without optional exercises)

| 1 | | Finger mobility 1<br>10 times | Page 29 |
|---|---|---|---|

| 2 | | Finger mobility 2<br>10 times (optional) | Page 30 |
|---|---|---|---|

| 19 | | Raising and lowering the shoulders<br>10 times (optional) | Page 46 |
|---|---|---|---|

| 12 | | Full arm rotations<br>10 times | Page 38 |
|---|---|---|---|

# CHAPTER FOUR

EXERCISES BY INSTRUMENT

| | | | |
|---|---|---|---|
| 20 | | Twisting the chest and arms<br>10 times (optional) | Page 46 |
| 32 | | Yes with the neck<br>10 times (optional) | Page 57 |
| 33 | | Maybe with the neck<br>10 times (optional) | Page 58 |
| 34 | | No with the neck<br>10 times | Page 59 |
| 37 | | Side of the neck<br>20" + 20" | Page 61 |
| 38 | | Scapula levator<br>20" + 20" | Page 61 |
| 35 | | Back of the neck<br>20" + 20" (optional) | Page 59 |
| 36 | | Front of the neck<br>20" + 20" | Page 60 |

| 14 | Fist out<br>20" + 20" | Page 40 |
|---|---|---|
| 16 | Hand back<br>20" + 20" | Page 42 |
| 21 | Chest<br>20" + 20" | Page 47 |
| 45 | Lower back<br>20" + 20" | Page 68 |
| 43 | Back<br>20" | Page 66 |
| 52 | Leg back 1<br>20" + 20" | Page 73 |
| 44 | Lateral abdominal muscles<br>20" + 20" | Page 67 |
| 23 | Latissimus dorsi<br>20" + 20" | Page 49 |

| CHAPTER FOUR | EXERCISES BY INSTRUMENT |

| 4 | 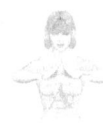 | Palm of the hand<br>20" | Page 31 |

## AFTER PLAYING

**Essential**
(6 minutes 20 seconds in total; 5 minutes 40 seconds without optional exercises)

| 37 | | Side of the neck<br>20" + 20" | Page 61 |

| 38 | | Scapula levator<br>20" + 20" | Page 61 |

| 35 | | Back of the neck<br>20" + 20" (optional) | Page 59 |

| 36 | | Front of the neck<br>20" + 20" | Page 60 |

| 15 | | Fist in<br>20" + 20" | Page 41 |

| 17 | | Hand down<br>20" + 20" | Page 42 |

**IN TUNE**

| 21 | | Chest<br>20" + 20" | Page 47 |
|---|---|---|---|
| 45 | | Lower back<br>20" + 20" | Page 68 |
| 43 | | Back<br>20" | Page 66 |
| 52 | | Leg back 1<br>20" + 20" | Page 73 |

## Complete
(8 minutes in total; 7 minutes 20 seconds without optional exercises)

| 37 | | Side of the neck<br>20" + 20" | Page 61 |
|---|---|---|---|
| 38 | | Scapula levator<br>20" + 20" | Page 61 |
| 35 | | Back of the neck<br>20" + 20" (optional) | Page 59 |

# CHAPTER FOUR

**EXERCISES BY INSTRUMENT**

| | | | |
|---|---|---|---|
| 36 | | Front of the neck<br>20" + 20" | Page 60 |
| 15 | | Fist in<br>20" + 20" | Page 41 |
| 17 | | Hand down<br>20" + 20" | Page 42 |
| 21 | | Chest<br>20" + 20" | Page 47 |
| 45 | | Lower back<br>20" + 20" | Page 68 |
| 43 | | Back<br>20" | Page 66 |
| 52 | | Leg back 1<br>20" + 20" | Page 73 |
| 44 | | Lateral abdominal muscles<br>20" + 20" | Page 67 |

| 23 | Latissimus dorsi 20" + 20" | Page 49 |
| 4 | Palm of the hand 20" | Page 31 |

# GROUP 14
# BRASS

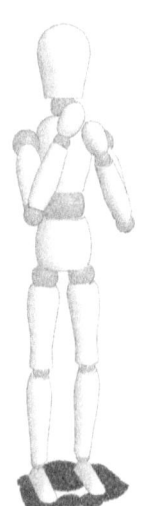

Musicians who play brass or similar instruments held in front of the body often stress the back in addition to the mouth region. They also tend to *close the shoulders*, sustaining them in a forward position that causes *dorsal hunching* and loss of the proper lumbar curve.

Incorporating specific exercises in the daily program to compensate for these imbalances is crucial in maintaining physical fitness and good health.

## BEFORE PLAYING

**Essential**
(8 minutes 10 seconds in total; 6 minutes without optional exercises)

| | | | |
|---|---|---|---|
| 1 | | Finger mobility 1<br>10 times (optional) | Page 29 |
| 12 | | Full arm rotations<br>10 times (optional) | Page 38 |
| 32 | | Yes with the neck<br>10 times (optional) | Page 57 |
| 33 | | Maybe with the neck<br>10 times (optional) | Page 58 |

| | | | |
|---|---|---|---|
| 34 | | No with the neck<br>10 times (optional) | Page 59 |
| 37 | | Side of the neck<br>20" + 20" | Page 61 |
| 38 | | Scapula levator<br>20" + 20" | Page 61 |
| 35 | | Back of the neck<br>20" + 20" (optional) | Page 59 |
| 36 | | Front of the neck<br>20" + 20" | Page 60 |
| 14 | | Fist out<br>20" + 20" | Page 40 |
| 16 | | Hand back<br>20" + 20" | Page 42 |
| 59 | | Vowels and consonants<br>30" | Page 79 |

**CHAPTER FOUR**                                                          EXERCISES BY INSTRUMENT

| | | | |
|---|---|---|---|
| 61 | | Two-sided face stretch<br>20" + 20" | Page 81 |
| 21 | | Chest<br>20" + 20" | Page 47 |
| 45 | | Lower back<br>20" + 20" | Page 68 |

**Complete**
(13 minutes 50 seconds in total; 8 minutes 40 seconds without optional exercises)

| | | | |
|---|---|---|---|
| 1 | | Finger mobility 1<br>10 times | Page 29 |
| 2 | | Finger mobility 2<br>10 times (optional) | Page 30 |
| 19 | | Raising and lowering the shoulders<br>10 times (optional) | Page 46 |
| 12 | | Full arm rotations<br>10 times | Page 38 |

# IN TUNE

| 20 | Twisting the chest and arms<br>10 times (optional) | Page 46 |
| 32 | Yes with the neck<br>10 times (optional) | Page 57 |
| 33 | Maybe with the neck<br>10 times (optional) | Page 58 |
| 34 | No with the neck<br>10 times | Page 59 |
| 37 | Side of the neck<br>20" + 20" | Page 61 |
| 38 | Scapula levator<br>20" + 20" | Page 61 |
| 35 | Back of the neck<br>20" + 20" (optional) | Page 59 |
| 36 | Front of the neck<br>20" + 20" | Page 60 |

# CHAPTER FOUR

EXERCISES BY INSTRUMENT

| | | | |
|---|---|---|---|
| 14 | | Fist out<br>20" + 20" | Page 40 |
| 15 | | Fist in<br>20" + 20" | Page 41 |
| 59 | | Vowels and consonants<br>30" | Page 79 |
| 60 | | One-sided face stretch<br>20" + 20" + 20" + 20" | Page 80 |
| 61 | | Two-sided face stretch<br>20" + 20" (optional) | Page 81 |
| 21 | | Chest<br>20" + 20" | Page 47 |
| 45 | | Lower back<br>20" + 20" | Page 68 |
| 4 | | Palm of the hand<br>20" | Page 31 |

# IN TUNE

| 3 |  | Hand muscles<br>20" + 20" + 20" + 20" (optional) | Page 31 |

| 44 | 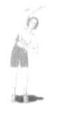 | Lower abdominal muscles<br>20" + 20" | Page 67 |

## AFTER PLAYING

**Essential**
(6 minutes in total; 5 minutes 20 seconds without optional exercises)

| 37 | | Side of the neck<br>20" + 20" | Page 61 |

| 38 | | Scapula levator<br>20" + 20" | Page 61 |

| 35 | | Back of the neck<br>20" + 20" (optional) | Page 59 |

| 36 | | Front of the neck<br>20" + 20" | Page 60 |

| 15 | | Fist in<br>20" + 20" | Page 41 |

| | | | |
|---|---|---|---|
| 17 | | Hand down<br>20" + 20" | Page 42 |
| 61 | | Two-sided face stretch<br>20" + 20" | Page 81 |
| 21 | | Chest<br>20" + 20" | Page 47 |
| 45 | | Lower back<br>20" + 20" | Page 68 |

**Complete**
(9 minutes 40 seconds in total; 7 minutes without optional exercises)

| | | | |
|---|---|---|---|
| 37 | | Side of the neck<br>20" + 20" | Page 61 |
| 38 | | Scapula levator<br>20" + 20" | Page 61 |
| 35 | | Back of the neck<br>20" + 20" (optional) | Page 59 |

| 36 | | Front of the neck<br>20" + 20" | Page 60 |
|---|---|---|---|
| 15 | | Fist in<br>20" + 20" | Page 41 |
| 17 | | Hand down<br>20" + 20" | Page 42 |
| 60 | | One-sided face stretch<br>20" + 20" + 20" + 20" | Page 80 |
| 61 | | Two-sided face stretch<br>20" + 20" (optional) | Page 81 |
| 21 | | Chest<br>20" + 20" | Page 47 |
| 45 | | Lower back<br>20" + 20" | Page 68 |
| 4 | | Palm of the hand<br>20" | Page 31 |

**CHAPTER FOUR**                          **EXERCISES BY INSTRUMENT**

| | | | |
|---|---|---|---|
| 3 | 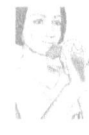 | Hand muscles<br>20" + 20" + 20" + 20" (optional) | Page 31 |
| 44 | 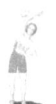 | Lower abdominal muscles<br>20" + 20" | Page 67 |

# GROUP 15
# BRASS, LATERAL

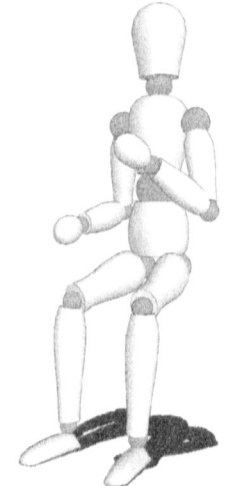

In addition to the demands on the face muscles, brass instruments that are played to the side or supported on the body often overstress the area around the spinal column.

Taking care of these muscles by means of a systematic program can help prevent future problems.

## BEFORE PLAYING

**Essential**
(8 minutes 30 seconds in total; 6 minutes 20 seconds without optional exercises)

| 1 | | Finger mobility 1<br>10 times (optional) | Page 29 |
|---|---|---|---|
| 12 | | Full arm rotations<br>10 times (optional) | Page 38 |
| 32 | | Yes with the neck<br>10 times (optional) | Page 57 |
| 33 | | Maybe with the neck<br>10 times (optional) | Page 58 |

# CHAPTER FOUR — EXERCISES BY INSTRUMENT

| # | | Exercise | Page |
|---|---|---|---|
| 34 | | No with the neck<br>10 times (optional) | Page 59 |
| 37 | | Side of the neck<br>20" + 20" | Page 61 |
| 38 | | Scapula levator<br>20" + 20" | Page 61 |
| 35 | | Back of the neck<br>20" + 20" (optional) | Page 59 |
| 36 | | Front of the neck<br>20" + 20" | Page 60 |
| 15 | | Fist in<br>20" + 20" | Page 41 |
| 17 | | Hand down<br>20" + 20" | Page 42 |
| 59 | | Vowels and consonants<br>30" | Page 79 |

**IN TUNE**

| 61 | Two-sided face stretch<br>20" + 20" | Page 81 |
| 23 | Latissimus dorsi<br>20" + 20" | Page 49 |
| 43 | Back<br>20" | Page 66 |
| 24 | Rear shoulder<br>20" + 20" | Page 50 |

## Complete
(13 minutes 10 seconds in total; 9 minutes 20 seconds without optional exercises)

| 1 | Finger mobility 1<br>10 times | Page 29 |
| 2 | Finger mobility 2<br>10 times (optional) | Page 30 |
| 19 | Raising and lowering the shoulders<br>10 times (optional) | Page 46 |

**CHAPTER FOUR** — EXERCISES BY INSTRUMENT

| | | | |
|---|---|---|---|
| 12 | | Full arm rotations<br>10 times | Page 38 |
| 20 | | Twisting the chest and arms<br>10 times (optional) | Page 46 |
| 32 | | Yes with the neck<br>10 times (optional) | Page 57 |
| 33 | | Maybe with the neck<br>10 times (optional) | Page 58 |
| 34 | | No with the neck<br>10 times | Page 59 |
| 37 | | Side of the neck<br>20" + 20" | Page 61 |
| 38 | | Scapula levator<br>20" + 20" | Page 61 |
| 35 | | Back of the neck<br>20" + 20" (optional) | Page 59 |

| 36 | | Front of the neck  20" + 20" | Page 60 |
|---|---|---|---|
| 15 | | Fist in  20" + 20" | Page 41 |
| 17 | | Hand down  20" + 20" | Page 42 |
| 59 | | Vowels and consonants  30" | Page 79 |
| 60 | | One-sided face stretch  20" + 20" + 20" + 20" | Page 80 |
| 61 | | Two-sided face stretch  20" + 20" (optional) | Page 81 |
| 23 | | Latissimus dorsi  20" + 20" | Page 49 |
| 43 | | Back  20" | Page 66 |

**CHAPTER FOUR**                        **EXERCISES BY INSTRUMENT**

| 24 | Rear shoulder 20" + 20" | Page 50 |
|----|-------------------------|---------|
| 39 | Interscapular 20" + 20" | Page 62 |
| 44 | Lower abdominal muscles 20" + 20" | Page 67 |

## AFTER PLAYING

**Essential**
(6 minutes 20 seconds in total; 5 minutes 40 seconds without optional exercises)

| 37 | Side of the neck 20" + 20" | Page 61 |
|----|----------------------------|---------|
| 38 | Scapula levator 20" + 20" | Page 61 |
| 35 | Back of the neck 20" + 20" (optional) | Page 59 |

**IN TUNE**

| 36 | | Front of the neck<br>20" + 20" | Page 60 |
| --- | --- | --- | --- |
| 14 | | Fist out<br>20" + 20" | Page 40 |
| 16 | | Hand back<br>20" + 20" | Page 42 |
| 61 | | Two-sided face stretch<br>20" + 20" | Page 81 |
| 23 | | Latissimus dorsi<br>20" + 20" | Page 49 |
| 43 | | Back<br>20" | Page 66 |
| 24 | | Rear shoulder<br>20" + 20" | Page 50 |

# CHAPTER FOUR — EXERCISES BY INSTRUMENT

## Complete
(9 minutes in total; 7 minutes 40 seconds without optional exercises)

| | | | |
|---|---|---|---|
| 37 | | Side of the neck<br>20" + 20" | Page 61 |
| 38 | | Scapula levator<br>20" + 20" | Page 61 |
| 35 | | Back of the neck<br>20" + 20" (optional) | Page 59 |
| 36 | | Front of the neck<br>20" + 20" | Page 60 |
| 14 | | Fist out<br>20" + 20" | Page 40 |
| 16 | | Hand back<br>20" + 20" | Page 42 |
| 60 | | One-sided face stretch<br>20" + 20" + 20" + 20" | Page 80 |

225

| | | | |
|---|---|---|---|
| 61 | | Two-sided face stretch<br>20" + 20" (optional) | Page 81 |
| 23 | | Latissimus dorsi<br>20" + 20" | Page 49 |
| 43 | | Back<br>20" | Page 66 |
| 24 | | Rear shoulder<br>20" + 20" | Page 50 |
| 39 | | Interscapular<br>20" + 20" | Page 62 |
| 44 | | Lower abdominal muscles<br>20" + 20 " | Page 67 |

Chapter Five

# STAYING HEALTHY AND FIT

A healthy and fit musician is capable of maintaining a steady pace of work without highs and lows, sustaining energy even on the harshest of days, tolerating the psychological stress of performing, and preserving equilibrium with regard to posture and tension.

Some musicians possess this state of fitness naturally and are able to maintain it without having to exercise. If you are not among these fortunate few, physical fitness can be achieved by two methods: the general aerobic workout (helpful for improving overall vitality and mood, as well as the ability to tolerate the physical and psychological stress from playing and performing) and the specialized workout (designed not only to improve overall physical condition before playing an instrument, but for daily life as well).

The general aerobic workout involves working the large muscle groups for a minimum of 30 minutes, two to three times a week. Running, walking at a brisk pace, swimming, dancing, bicycling, rowing, or skating, among other activities, are all considered aerobic workouts.

Every musician should discover what aerobic activity works best for them. Consider the following factors: convenience (it does not make sense to swim if the closest swimming pool is an hour away), body type (it is not advantageous for an overweight musician to run, since it will overstress the knees and ankles; in this case, it would be better ride a bike), and complementary instrumental posture (the posture required to play an instrument should not be the same as that required by the activity, as shown in the following figures).

# CHAPTER FIVE

STAYING HEALTHY AND FIT

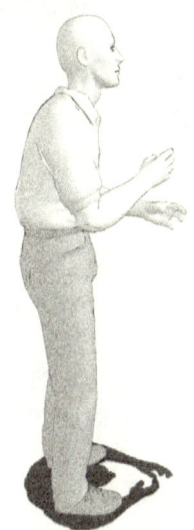
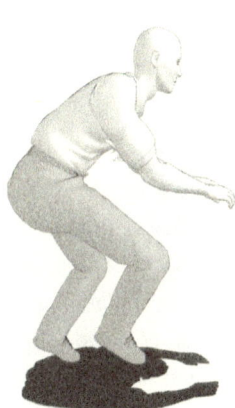

*A clarinetist whose playing posture involves a sustained forward position of the shoulders, a hunched thoracic region, and a curved neck would not receive the maximum benefit from cycling since a similar posture is used.*

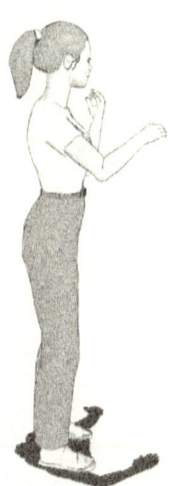
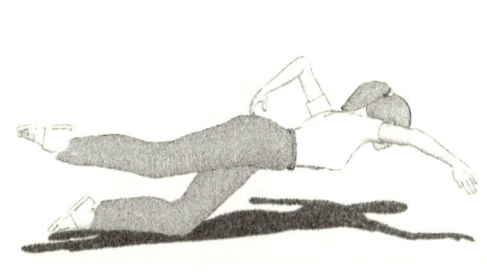

*It would also not be advisable for a violinist, who tends to overly curve the lower part of the spinal column and excessively tense the shoulders, to swim the front crawl or breaststroke since these strokes utilize similar postures.*

It seems obvious that it would be better for the clarinetist to decide on swimming and the violinist on cycling.

The specialized workout can be achieved with a set of stretches and muscle strengthening exercises. These are totally independent of the before and after playing programs (warm-up and cool-down) and are not meant to be a replacement. The warm-up and cool-down exercises are done with regard to instrumental activity and have been designed to prepare for and recover from the physical and psychological stresses of playing. These should be always done whenever the instrument is played. The specialized workouts aim to maintain the body in the best possible condition and include muscle strengthening programs for zones such as the hands, arms, shoulders, and back.

Two types of specialized workout programs have been designed to facilitate follow-through. The essential program, or short program (about 20 minutes in duration), is designed for musicians who do not have a lot of time to devote to workouts, those who require a transition period by starting with an easier workout, or those who have never worked out or are not accustomed to working out. The complete program (about one hour in duration) provides a more comprehensive workout.

Any training or physical conditioning program is based on consistent performance of an exercise regimen. A minimum workout frequency (at least three days a week) and regularity (not skipping too many days in a row) must be maintained. However, it is not necessary to do the complete program every day. You can alternate complete and essential programs every other day.

Since none of the exercises being proposed entail significant strain on the muscles, it is not necessary to schedule days off for recovery, as is generally done in strengthening programs. However, if a musician expects a hard day of concerts, rehearsals, classes, or other physical activities, it might be better to only do the part of the program that involves stretching.

# CHAPTER FIVE                                           STAYING HEALTHY AND FIT

## Essential Program
(32 minutes 30 seconds in total; 23 minutes 20 seconds without optional exercises)

| 1  | | Finger mobility 1<br>10 times (optional)     | Page 29 |
|----|---|----------------------------------------------|---------|
| 12 | | Full arm rotations<br>10 times (optional)    | Page 38 |
| 32 | | Yes with the neck<br>10 times (optional)     | Page 57 |
| 33 | | Maybe with the neck<br>10 times (optional)   | Page 58 |
| 34 | | No with the neck<br>10 times (optional)      | Page 59 |
| 37 | | Side of the neck<br>20" + 20" (optional)     | Page 61 |
| 38 | | Scapula levator<br>20" + 20" (optional)      | Page 61 |

## IN TUNE

| 36 | | Front of the neck  20" + 20" (optional) | Page 60 |
| 35 | | Back of the neck  20" + 20" (optional) | Page 59 |
| 14 | | Fist out  20" + 20" (optional) | Page 40 |
| 16 | | Hand back  20" + 20" (optional) | Page 42 |
| 52 | | Leg back 1  20" + 20" | Page 73 |
| 46 | | Spinal twist  20" + 20" | Page 68 |
| 40 | | Flexing the lumbar spine  20" x 2 | Page 64 |
| 47 | | Front hip area  20" + 20" | Page 69 |

# CHAPTER FIVE — STAYING HEALTHY AND FIT

| | | | |
|---|---|---|---|
| 54 | | Glutes<br>20" + 20" | Page 75 |
| 41 | | Child's pose<br>20" x 3 | Page 65 |
| 50 | | Abdominal workout using a wall<br>10" x 6 x 3 | Page 71 |
| 51 | | Hamstrings and abdominals<br>10" x 6 | Page 72 |
| 7 | | Picking up marbles<br>3' | Page 34 |
| 9 | | Rubber bands<br>3' | Page 35 |
| 25 | | Pillow<br>6" x 15 + 6" x 15 | Page 50 |
| 28 | | Back to the wall<br>6" x 15 + 6" x 15 | Page 53 |

**IN TUNE**

29 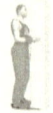 Pectoral to the wall  Page 53
 6" x 15 + 6" x 15

# CHAPTER FIVE — STAYING HEALTHY AND FIT

## Essential Program: Wind Instruments
(additional 5 minutes, 50 seconds)

Wind instrumentalists should add the following specialized exercises for the zone around the mouth to supplement the essential program.

| 61 | Two-sided face stretch  20" + 20" | Page 81 |
|---|---|---|
| 59 | Vowels and consonants  30" | Page 79 |
| 62 | Straight smile  6" x 5 | Page 81 |
| 63 | Sneer  6" x 5 + 6" x 5 | Page 82 |
| 64 | Kiss  6" x 5 | Page 83 |
| 65 | Fish  6" x 5 | Page 83 |

## IN TUNE

| | | | |
|---|---|---|---|
| 66 | | Shivers<br>6" x 5 | Page 84 |
| 67 | | Upwards smile<br>6" x 5 | Page 84 |
| 68 | | Frown<br>6" x 5 | Page 85 |
| 61 | | Two-sided face stretch<br>20" + 20" | Page 81 |

## Complete Program

(55 minutes 50 seconds in total; 46 minutes 40 seconds without optional exercises)

| 1 | | Finger mobility 1<br>10 times (optional) | Page 29 |
|---|---|---|---|
| 12 | | Full arm rotations<br>10 times (optional) | Page 38 |
| 32 | | Yes with the neck<br>10 times (optional) | Page 57 |
| 33 | | Maybe with the neck<br>10 times (optional) | Page 58 |
| 34 | | No with the neck<br>10 times (optional) | Page 59 |
| 37 | | Side of the neck<br>20" + 20" (optional) | Page 61 |
| 38 | | Scapula levator<br>20" + 20" (optional) | Page 61 |

| | | | |
|---|---|---|---|
| 36 | | Front of the neck<br>20" + 20" (optional) | Page 60 |
| 35 | | Back of the neck<br>20" + 20" (optional) | Page 59 |
| 14 | | Fist out<br>20" + 20" (optional) | Page 40 |
| 16 | | Hand back<br>20" + 20" (optional) | Page 42 |
| 52 | | Leg back I<br>20" + 20" | Page 73 |
| 46 | | Spinal twist<br>20" + 20" | Page 68 |
| 42 | | Straightening the lumbar curve on the ground<br>10" x 3 | Page 66 |
| 40 | | Flexing the lumbar spine<br>20" x 2 | Page 64 |

# CHAPTER FIVE  STAYING HEALTHY AND FIT

| 18 | Hand inclined 20" + 20" | Page 43 |
| --- | --- | --- |
| 48 | Rectus abdominals 6" x 10 + 6" x 10 | Page 70 |
| 49 | Oblique abdominals 6" x 10 + 6" x 10 | Page 70 |
| 50 | Abdominal workout using a wall 10" x 6 x 3 | Page 71 |
| 51 | Hamstrings and abdominals 10" x 6 | Page 72 |
| 56 | Internal leg 2 20" | Page 76 |
| 47 | Front hip area 20" x 20" | Page 69 |
| 55 | Internal leg 1 20" x 20" | Page 76 |

# IN TUNE

| 57 | | Front leg  
20" x 20" | Page 77 |
|---|---|---|---|
| 58 | | Calf muscles  
20" x 20" | Page 78 |
| 7 | | Picking up marbles  
3' | Page 34 |
| 8 | | Intrinsic plus  
3' | Page 34 |
| 9 | | Rubber bands  
3' | Page 35 |
| 10 | | Ball juggling  
3' | Page 36 |
| 11 | | Ping-pong balls  
3' | Page 37 |
| 25 | | Pillow  
6" x 15 + 6" x 15 | Page 50 |

| CHAPTER FIVE | | | STAYING HEALTHY AND FIT |
|---|---|---|---|
| 26 | | Chair<br>6" x 15 | Page 61 |
| 27 | | Pole back<br>3' | Page 52 |
| 28 | | Back to the wall<br>6" x 15 + 6" x 15 | Page 53 |
| 29 | | Pectoral to the wall<br>6" x 15 + 6" x 15 | Page 53 |
| 30 | | Back with elastic band<br>3" x 20 + 3" x 20 | Page 54 |
| 31 | | Pectoral elastic band<br>3" x 20 + 3" x 20 | Page 55 |

**IN TUNE**

**Essential Program: Wind Instruments**
(additional 8 minutes 30 seconds in total; 5 minutes 50 seconds without optional exercises)

---

Wind instrumentalists should add the following specialized exercises for the zone around the mouth to supplement the complete program:

| 60 | One-sided face stretch<br>20" + 20" + 20" + 20" (optional) | Page 80 |
|---|---|---|
| 61 | Two-sided face stretch<br>20" + 20" | Page 81 |
| 59 | Vowels and consonants<br>30" | Page 79 |
| 62 | Straight smile<br>6" x 5 | Page 81 |
| 63 | Sneer<br>6" x 5 + 6" x 5 | Page 82 |
| 64 | Kiss<br>6" x 5 | Page 83 |

**CHAPTER FIVE**             **STAYING HEALTHY AND FIT**

| 65 | | Fish<br>6" x 5 | Page 83 |
|---|---|---|---|
| 66 | | Shivers<br>6" x 5 | Page 84 |
| 67 | | Upward smile<br>6" x 5 | Page 84 |
| 68 | | Frown<br>6" x 5 | Page 85 |
| 61 | | Two-sided face stretch<br>20" + 20" | Page 81 |
| 60 | | One-sided face stretch<br>20" + 20" + 20" + 20" (optional) | Page 80 |

Chapter Six

# EXERCISES FOR SPECIAL SITUATIONS

Doing physical conditioning exercises before and after playing should be a routine as natural to a musician as tuning the instrument, adding rosin to the bow, removing water from the valve slides, or adjusting the reed. In addition, experience has shown that getting into the habit of stretching during rehearsals or concerts is one of the best tools a musician has to prevent injuries and perform their best.

However, the conditions under which musicians must perform are not always the best for doing exercises. Often the main limitation of exercising is the fear of what one's colleagues or director might think. Also, some musicians might find it difficult to exercise while sitting down or holding an instrument in their hands.

However, once the basic technique of performing a stretching exercise in optimum conditions has been mastered, then it should not be too hard to adapt that exercise to situations that are less than ideal.

To make this easier, here are some examples of how stretching exercises can be adapted so they can be done in special situations. The goal is for musicians to be able to find the best way to adapt all exercises that are considered useful so that they can be performed correctly regardless of the conditions.

# CHAPTER SIX

EXERCISES FOR SPECIAL SITUATIONS

## 1 Adaptation of the "hand-back" exercise

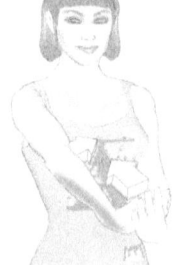

Stretching the finger flexor muscles is one of the most important stretches for any musician. The problem is that during a rehearsal or concert, despite breaks, having to hold an instrument makes it difficult to do these exercises.

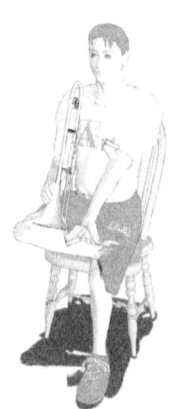

One alternative would be to use the opposite leg crossed over the other as a support. This leaves one hand free to hold the instrument.

Another option is placing your hand under your buttock with the palm facing the chair. Pianists can sit on both hands at the same time. The more you *extend your elbow*, the higher the level of stretch.

## 2 Adaptation of the "wrist-down" exercise

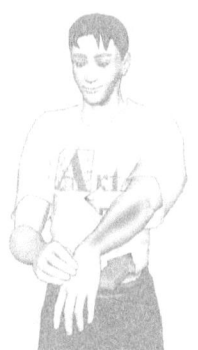

Your chair can also be used to do other stretching exercises, like those for the *extensor digitorum profundus*[7] of the fingers and wrist.

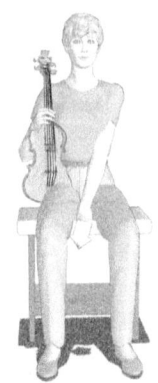

Put the back of your hand on your chair, between your legs, with the fingertips facing you. With your *elbow fully extended*, press downward, trying to *flex your wrist* as much as possible, but as with all stretches, avoiding pain. You can also do this stretch with your fist closed, *flexing the fingers*.

Maintain pressure for 20 seconds; this exercise can be repeated as many times as needed.

## 3  Adaptation of the "thumb-back" exercise

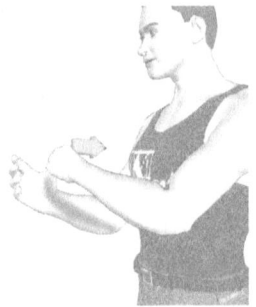

Many instrumentalists use their thumb intensely (woodwind instruments, plucked and bowed string instruments, etc.). For them, it is crucial to relieve thumb stress. Stretching exercises can help minimize the effects of these stresses. These exercises will be all the more effective if they are done not only before and after playing, but also during the short breaks between playing.

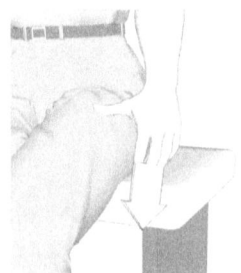

One adaptation to be able to do this exercise under these circumstances is to support the thumb on your leg or on the edge of the chair, allowing you to *extend your thumb up* while pushing the hand and entire arm downward.

## 4  Adaptations for neck stretches

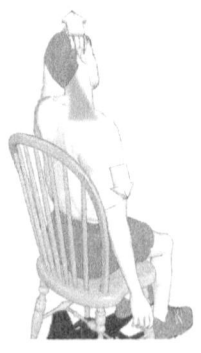

As previously mentioned, the neck and back area tends to accumulate more stress in musicians. In addition to possibly causing discomfort, this can often imperceptibly lead to a suboptimal performance.

Any of the stretching exercises for the neck area can easily be adapted for implementation under any circumstance. In order for these to be effective, you need to be aware of the part of the body being stretched. Be sure to relax that area and try to separate the two ends of the muscle, which in this case is achieved by dropping the shoulder.

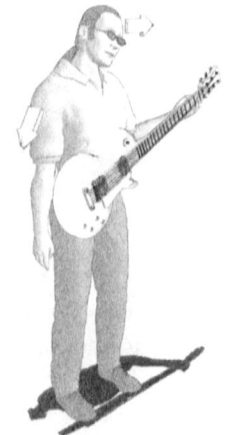

As an example, in order to stretch your *trapezius muscle*[34], it is not enough for you to bend your neck to the opposite side. You should also lower your shoulder.

One way to completely and simply stretch a large portion of the neck muscles is the clock exercise.

# CHAPTER SIX

EXERCISES FOR SPECIAL SITUATIONS

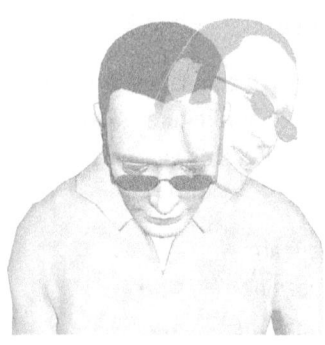

*The figure shows the position of the head in two intermediate points of the clock exercise, at 6 o'clock and at 3 o'clock.*

Begin by bending your neck forward, trying to touch your chin to your chest, releasing tension and stretching the muscles of the back part of the neck (mainly the *splenius muscle*[32]). Hold this position for at least five seconds and then *tilt your head* slightly to the right and stop for at least five seconds more in the new position. If you think of the initial position as your head being at 6 o'clock, the new position will be at 7 o'clock. Here and in the following position at 8 o'clock, the *trapezius*[34] and *scapula levator*[29] are being worked. Move your head in a similar manner, stopping at each hour position of a clock for a minimum of five seconds until you reach 9 o'clock. In this position the ear is almost touching your shoulder and your chin is up, stretching the *sternocleidomastoid*[33]. From there, move in a similar manner back towards 6 o'clock and continue until you reach 3 o'clock. Only move from shoulder to shoulder. Do not allow your head to go back past 3 o'clock or 9 o'clock.

## 5   Adaptations of shoulder and neck stretching exercises

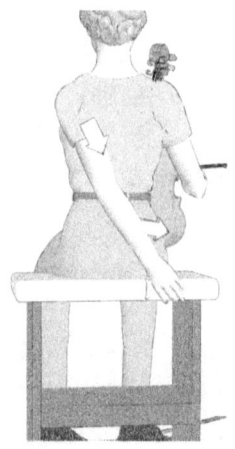

Your chair can also be used as an effective substitute for the function usually performed by the arm opposite the one being stretched.

One possibility is to lean forward in your chair, putting one arm behind you and grabbing the support bar or the edge of the seat on the opposite side. This makes it possible to more efficiently lower your shoulder and stretch your neck and shoulder muscles.

Another possibility is to lower your shoulder by grabbing the leg of the chair on the same side you wish to stretch.

## 6  Adaptations of the "chest" stretching exercise

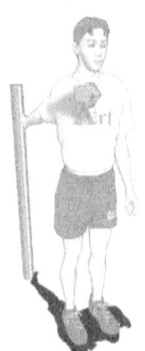

Undoubtedly the best way to stretch the torso and arm muscles is in a door frame or by grabbing a piece of furniture. When you are sufficiently trained, this can be done sitting down in the same chair in which you are playing.

This exercise involves putting your arm over the back of the chair and leaning your entire torso forward.

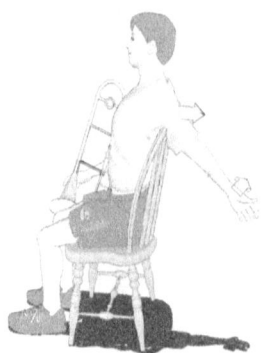

In order for this exercise to be more effective and to avoid causing problems in other areas, you must be careful not to twist your spine or increase your lumbar spine curvature (*lordosis*).

## 7  Adaptation of the "spinal twist" exercise

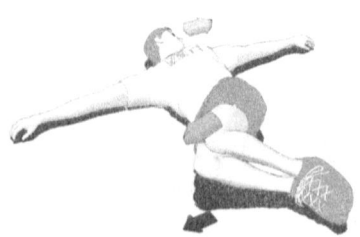

Sitting down for long periods of time, especially when you are being subjected to stress, usually leads to a certain degree of discomfort around the lower part of the spinal column.

You can significantly reduce this tension by doing exercise *46-Spinal twist*. This exercise is generally done on the floor, but it can also be done without getting up from your chair.

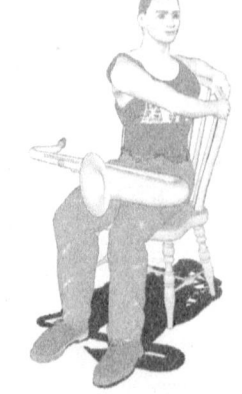

Turn your torso to the left or right and try to grab the back of your chair with both hands, pulling to twist your spine.

As with most stretches, it is important to keep your breathing relaxed. Relaxed breathing is even more important in this exercise since the twisting may depend on how full of air your chest is.

Chapter Seven

# EXERCISES THAT ARE ADVISED AGAINST

Just as not all sports are recommended for all people, not all exercises are suitable for all musicians.

Although used for many years, some exercises have been demonstrated to be dangerous to different areas of the body. This has gradually led to the acceptance that these exercises are no longer recommended for anyone.

On the other hand, some exercises may be good for most people, but might be considered too taxing for areas of the body that already tend to be over-stressed in musicians.

The exercises included in the workout programs within this book have been carefully selected with the criterion that they not cause any type of injury. However, a musician may have learned or been previously advised to do an exercise without being sure if it were suitable.

Since it is impossible to provide an exhaustive description of all of these exercises, the most common ones have been analyzed so musicians can identify those that might be harmful.

# CHAPTER SEVEN

**EXERCISES THAT ARE ADVISED AGAINST**

## 1 Neck hyperflexion exercises

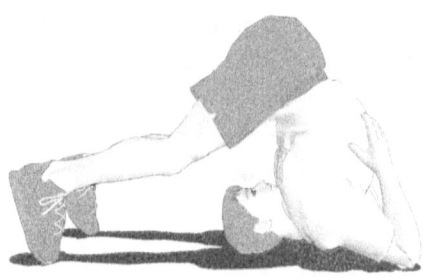

Although it is important for a musician to relieve stress in the neck and back, caution must be taken in order to prevent other areas of the body from being injured or stressed when stretching. An example of this is an exercise that requires an excessive *flexing* of the cervical column. This occurs when the exercise is done under a heavy load, as shown in the figure.

Besides causing dizziness, these types of exercises place significant stress on the vertebral discs, harm the small joints that stabilize the spinal column, and tend to compress the nerve endings in that area. Even a musician who has never had neck problems should avoid this type of exercise.

If you want to stretch the muscles in the back of the neck, simply *bend your head (flexion)* and try to touch your chin to your chest. If you want to intensify the stretch, you can press your head down with your hands, being careful not to exert excessive pressure.

## 2 Hyperextension exercises of the cervical column

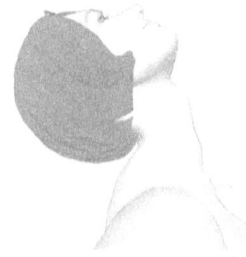

The movement of *extending the neck*, even when done smoothly, can be harmful if certain limits are exceeded.

In addition to muscles, the stability of the spine comes from the bone support provided by the vertebrae and small joints located in the back of the neck.

These joints are pinched when you *extend your neck* beyond 45° to the vertical.

As explained in the flexibility exercise *32-Yes with the neck* (page 57), in order to obtain proper *extension*, limit your movement to the point where, without moving your eyes, you start to see the ceiling just above your head. Always stay within this limit. This proper *extension* protects the area and prevents harming the joints, intervertebral discs, and cervical nerves.

## 3 Cervical circumduction

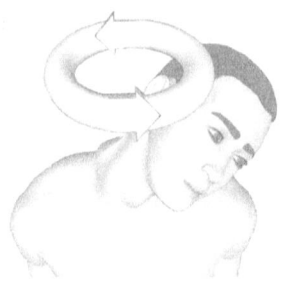

When any type of movement is made with the spine, the small joints that provide stability to the vertebrae slide with respect to their adjacent joints. Right next to this area are nerves that originate in the spine and are directed to the various parts of the body to capture sensory stimuli and send motor orders.

Some movements can cause these joints to be pinched, resulting in a noticeable shrinking of the space through which the nerves pass. One such movement is the complete rotation of the head (called circumduction). It is recommended that this exercise never be done by anyone, much less musicians in whom the cervical area is often subject to significant stress.

When doing a head rotation, initiate it to the right side without entirely reaching the midpoint behind your head (chin to the sky). The rotation is then reversed until you reach the midpoint in the front (chin to the chest) and continued to the left side.

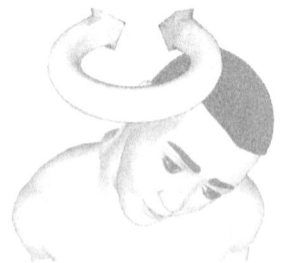

*Partial rotations can be done.*

## 4 Lumbar hyperextensions

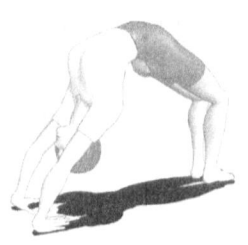

Lumbar hyperextensions are a set of exercises that, although considered beneficial for some people, can lead to excessive stress or risks to a musician's health. These exercises notably include: the hyperextension with four points of support (known as the bridge), the hyperextension with eccentric contractions of the abdominal muscles (passing the ball backwards overhead while on your knees), face down lumbar toning exercises (forming a boat with your feet off the ground or a reverse crunch with someone holding down your feet), the coxofemoral hyperextension (on all fours, raising one leg above horizontal), and standing with your arms back and accentuating the lumbar curve.

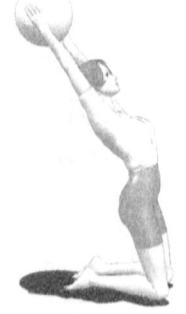

# CHAPTER SEVEN

## EXERCISES THAT ARE ADVISED AGAINST

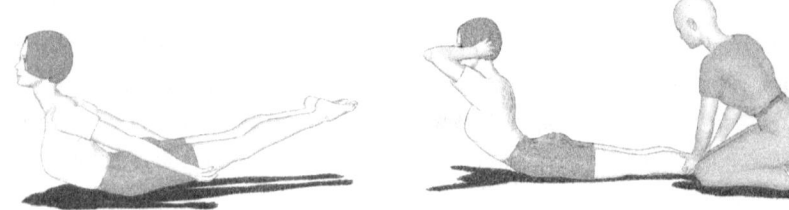

All of these exercises can cause excessive strain on the nerves, blood vessels, joints of the vertebrae, and nucleus pulposus of the vertebral disc.

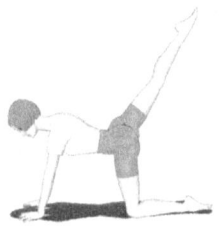

Although it is possible to do these exercises without negative effects, they will most likely eventually cause problems affecting a musician's quality of life.

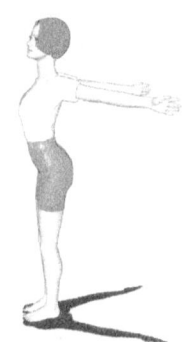

### 5   Some abdominal exercises

Although toning of the abdominal muscles is essential in maintaining a healthy spine, some exercises can be counterproductive. These include exercises that cause excessive stress to the lumbar discs or create hyperextension of the spinal column.

Two examples of this are lifting your torso up from the waist (doing full sit-ups) and raising your legs straight up from the ground.

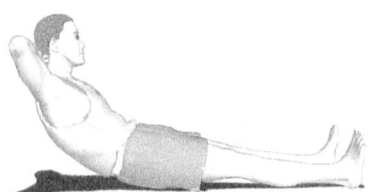
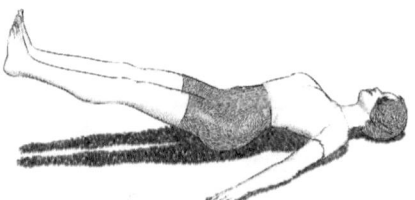

To avoid the problems these exercises can cause, a musician should tone the abdominal muscles by keeping their *knees bent* at all times (exercises *48-Rectus abdominals*, page 70, and *49-Oblique abdominals*, page 70), utilizing positions that reduce the lumbar *lordosis* (*50-Abdominal workout using a wall*, page 71, or *51-Hamstrings and abdominals*, page 72), or by raising only the upper part of the torso (crunches).

## 6  Hyperflexion of the lumbar column

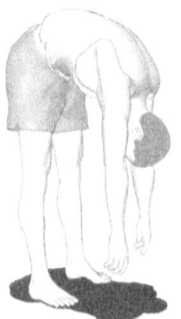

For many years, toe-touches have been a traditional exercise to work the elasticity of the spine and legs. However, this exercise simultaneously stretches numerous muscles which in turn generates a high amount of stress in the lumbar column. This can mean a significant risk of injury to the vertebral discs and the ligaments that stabilize the area. In addition, it is difficult to ensure a balanced and beneficial muscular workout.

A better alternative is to stretch the spinal area and the *hamstrings*[ll] separately (exercises *52-Leg back 1*, page 73, *53-Leg back 2*, page 74, *45-Lower back*, page 68, and *46-Spinal twist*, page 68), or do toe-touches with the *knees bent* and without trying to touch the floor with your hands. This simply involves letting the body, arms, and head fall forward, observing the stretch in the back part of the *hamstrings*[ll] and in the shoulders.

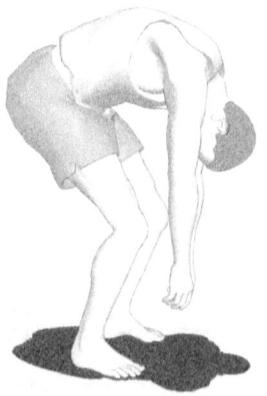

*This exercise can be done while maintaining bent knees.*

## Appendix

# GLOSSARY OF MUSCLES

It is evident that musicians can play perfectly well without any knowledge of anatomy. However, it can be useful to have a basic understanding of the subject, either for the purpose of better apprehension of how movements are executed and gestures are maintained, or to comprehend which muscles are used to compensate for stress in a given area.

Not all muscles of the human anatomy, or even all muscles used by musicians, are included in this glossary. It only includes the most important muscles and those cited throughout the book.

For each muscle listed, information is provided regarding location, function, examples of how it is used when playing music, and corresponding exercises to work the muscle. It should be noted that only some instruments are cited in the examples to facilitate the understanding of a muscle's function. This does not imply that the muscle is not used when playing other instruments.

The technical terms that appear in italics throughout the book are explained here in the glossary.

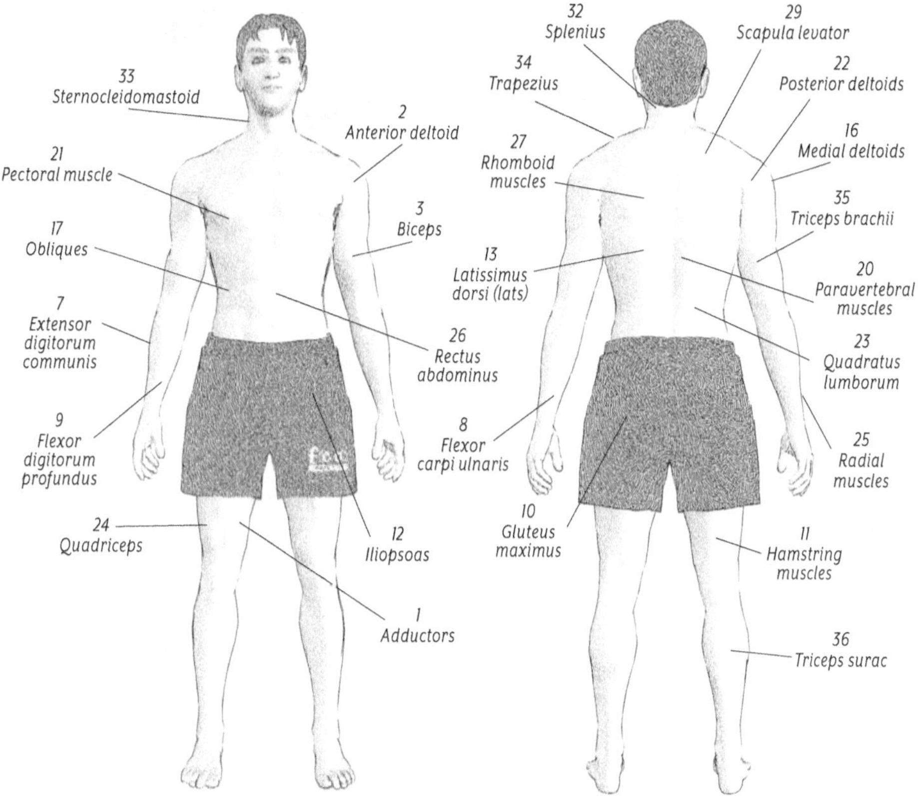

# APPENDIX A

## GLOSSARY OF MUSCLES

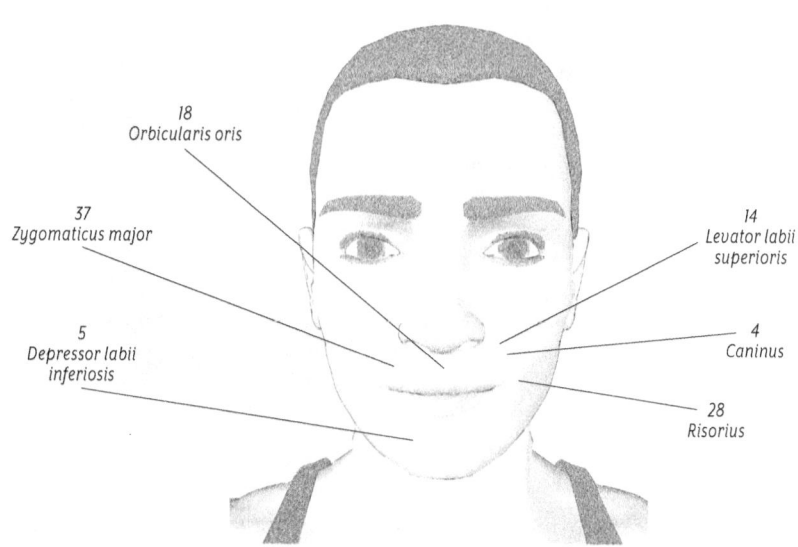

# IN TUNE

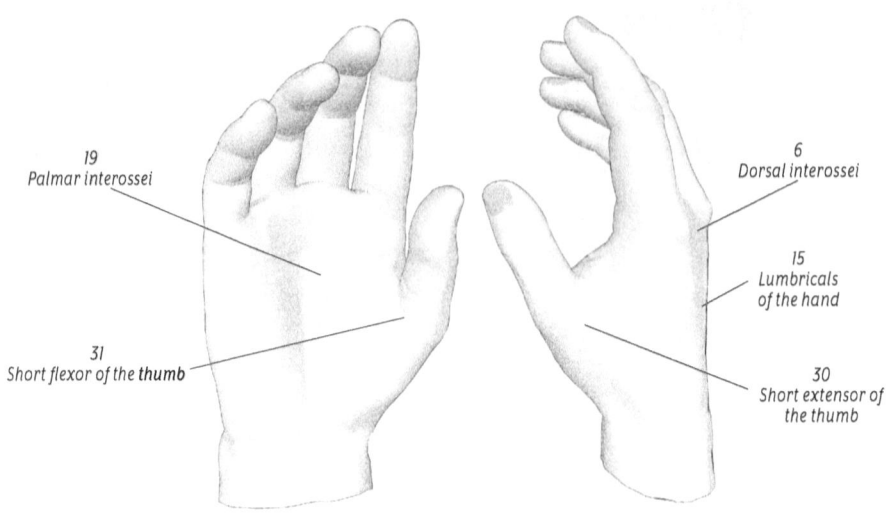

19 Palmar interossei
31 Short flexor of the thumb
6 Dorsal interossei
15 Lumbricals of the hand
30 Short extensor of the thumb

## 1 Adductors

This set is formed by five muscles that occupy the inner part of the thigh. They are the pectineus, adductor minimus, adductor brevis, adductor longus, and adductor magnus.

**Location:** The adductors originate in the pubis, from the highest point to the ischiopubic ramus, and are inserted into the femur.

**Function:** They perform adduction; i.e., bringing the leg to the centerline of the body.

**Example:** This set of muscles creates the movement of bringing the knees together which makes it possible to hold certain instruments including percussion (e.g., bongos) and cello. Since the adductors help stabilize the leg when they work in conjunction with the *quadriceps*[24], musicians who simultaneously engage their arms and legs utilize them. For example, when a harpist moves the pedals to change the

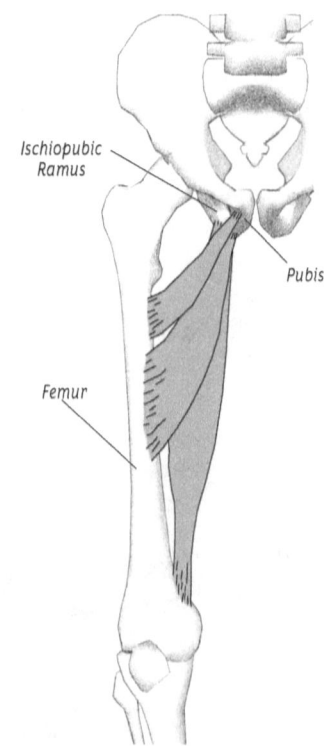

Ischiopubic Ramus
Pubis
Femur

pitch, the leg is stabilized by these muscles when going from the upper to the medium and lower positions.

**Exercise:** Even though these muscles are not usually overstressed, most musicians benefit from stretching these muscles to maintain a good balance in that part of the body. Stretching exercises for the adductors are *55-Internal leg 1* (page 76) and *56-Internal leg 2* (page 76).

## 2  Anterior deltoid

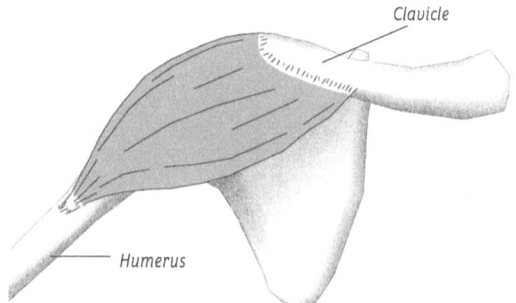

**Location:** The anterior deltoid originates from the lateral third of the clavicle and inserts in the external upper arm, on the outer part of the humerus, at the deltoid tuberosity along with the other two heads of the deltoids (*medial*[16] and (*posterior*[22]).

**Function:** The anterior deltoid allows *flexion* of the shoulder joint (by moving the arm forward) and creates the *internal rotation of the arm* when you are lying on your back. It also contributes to the stabilization of the shoulder.

**Example:** Most wind musicians (e.g., clarinetists, trumpet players, and oboists) utilize the anterior deltoid when moving their arms forward to support their instrument. Percussionists also use it when bringing mallets or drum sticks to their instrument, as do harpists in order to hold their arms at the strings.

**Exercise:** Any musician who plays with their arms forward and raised should do the stretching exercise *21-Chest* (page 47).

## 3  Biceps

**Location:** This muscle consists of two muscle sets called the long head and the short head. The long head originates in the glenoid cavity of the shoulder blade, and the short head in the coracoid process. The two muscle sets join and run through the front of the arm, ending in the radial tuberosity and expanding to the flexor muscles fascia.

**Function:** Although the biceps also act on the movement of the shoulder (primarily contributing to antepulsion), their basic function is the *flexion of the elbow* and the *external rotation* of the forearm.

**Example:** All musicians who play instruments that must be held with their hands, especially if the *elbow is bent* (such as the clarinet, trumpet, harmonica, or cymbals), use the biceps on a continuous basis (isometrically). Keep in mind that isometric contraction is what most easily causes fatigue and muscular overload.

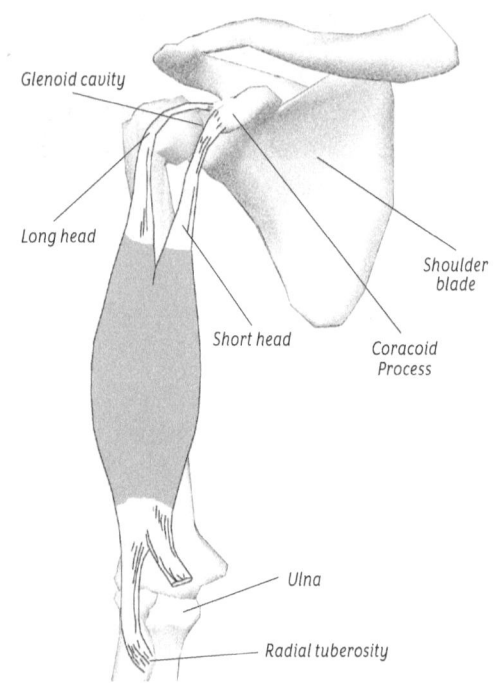

Other musicians use the biceps more dynamically (repetitions of contraction and relaxation). One example is how string players use their bows. When the tip of the bow is on the string, you almost fully *extend your elbow*. When the frog of the bow is on the string, you significantly *bend your elbow*. During the movement from tip to frog, the biceps are contracted. The muscle then partially relaxes when traveling back to the tip.

Another example of dynamic use is when harpists *bend their elbows* to reach the high notes that are closer to the body, or when trombone players shorten and extend their slides by *bending* and *straightening their elbows*..

**Exercise:** *21-Chest* (page 47) can be helpful in stretching the biceps.

## 4  Caninus

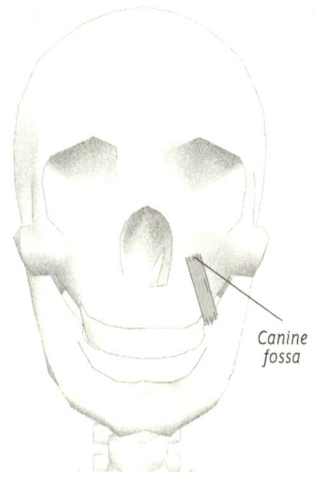

*Canine fossa*

**Location:** The caninus arises from the canine fossa and ends at the corner of the mouth.

**Function:** It deepens the lateral groove from the nose to the side of the mouth.

**Example:** As all the muscles of the mouth area are interconnected, the caninus is used by all wind musicians. The most specific action of this muscle is laughing or sneering.

**Exercise:** To make this and the other muscles of the mouth more flexible, *59-Vowels and consonants* (page 79) may be worthwhile. Exercise *63-Sneer* (page 82) is useful for toning this area.

## 5  Depressor labii inferioris

**Location:** The depressor labii inferioris arises from the oblique line of the lower jawbone (in the chin) to the fibers of the lower lip, intermixing with the *orbicularis oris*[18].

**Function:** It directs the lower lip and the corner of the mouth downward and outward, tensing the skin.

**Example:** As all the muscles of the mouth area are interconnected, the depressor labii inferioris is used by all wind musicians. The most specific gesture of this muscle is shivering.

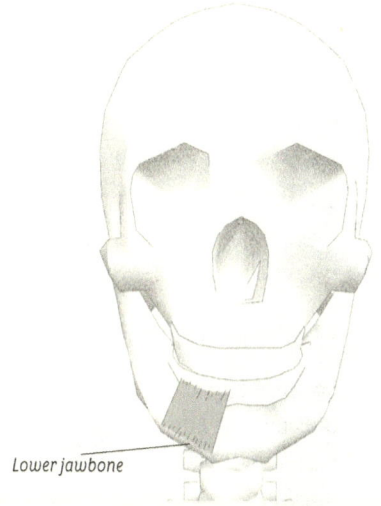

*Lower jawbone*

**Exercise:** To make this and the other muscles of the mouth more flexible, *59-Vowels and consonants* (page 79) may be worthwhile. *66-Shivers* (page 84) is useful for toning this area.

## 6 Dorsal interossei

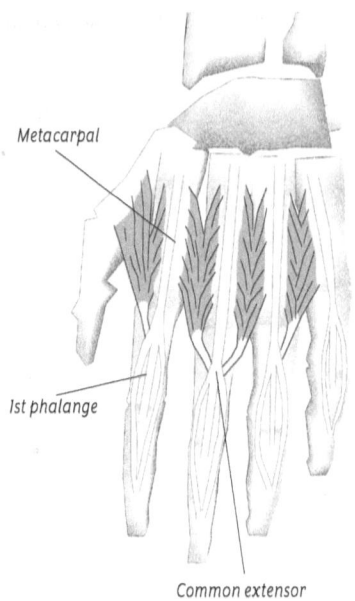

*Metacarpal*

*1st phalange*

*Common extensor*

**Location:** These are four small muscles in the back of the hand that originate from the inner borders of the metacarpal bones and are inserted into the base of the first phalanges and the tendon of the *extensor digitorum communis*[19].

**Function:** The dorsal interossei muscles separate the index, middle, and ring fingers as well as assist in their *flexion*. In addition, the first dorsal interossei helps to bring the thumb closer to the palm.

**Example:** When a cellist uses finger extensions, the dorsal interossei muscles aid in separating the index and middle fingers. The same happens when opening the hand to make octaves or ninths on the cello or piano.

**Exercise:** If these muscles are weak, the ability to open the fingers is reduced. Accordingly, to improve strength, rather than forcing the separation between fingers with the opposing hand or external devices, it is better to tone these muscles with exercises *7-Picking up marbles* (page 34), *8-Intrinsic plus* (page 34), *9-Rubber bands* (page 35), and *10-Ball juggling* (page 36). Flexibility can be improved with *1-Finger mobility 1* (page 29) and stretching with *3-Hand muscles* (page 31).

## 7 Extensor digitorum communis

**Location:** The extensor digitorum communis originates from the lateral epicondyle of the humerus and goes down through the back part of the forearm. It forms four terminal tendons that are directed to the fingers (not the thumb) and inserted in the base of the second and third phalanges.

**Function:** This muscle *extends* the *metacarpophalangeal joints* of the last four fingers and, together with the *lumbricals of the hand*[15] and *palmar interossei*[19], allows for the *extension* of the *interphalangeal joints* of the fingers. The extensor digitorum communis also contributes to the separation of the index, ring, and middle fingers as well as the *extension of the wrist*.

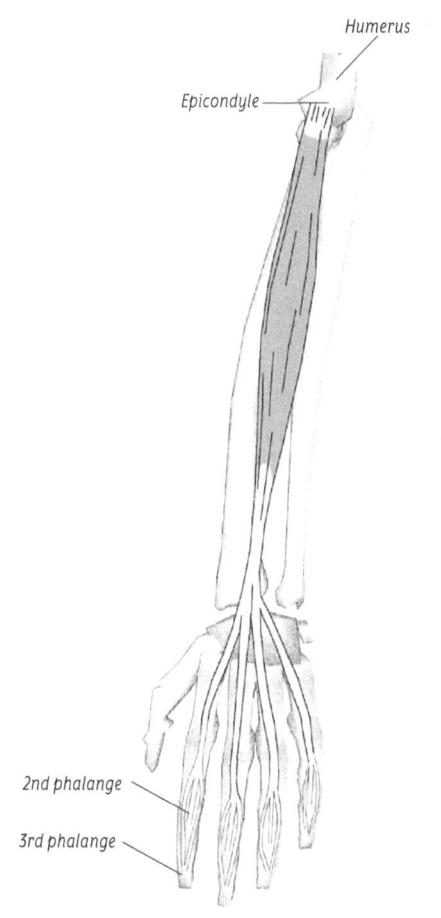

Humerus
Epicondyle
2nd phalange
3rd phalange

**Example:** This muscle works whenever musicians raise their fingers from the keys, buttons, pistons, or holes. It is also actuated when holding the fingers in the air in preparation to play. Since all fingers do not have their own muscles (flexors or extensors), the mind must learn to activate, in a more or less isolated manner, only a part of these muscles in order to move the fingers independently. When a pianist plays a 2-3 combination trill (index and middle finger), the part of the flexor that corresponds to the index finger is first contracted. As this relaxes, the pianist begins to contract the part of the flexor corresponding to the middle finger. This continues on in an alternating fashion.

**Exercise:** The extensor digitorum communis performs two functions. The more visible is that of moving the fingers. It also helps to stabilize the fingers and the wrist. Combining these two tasks, for long periods of time and with speed, involves a high level of stress. Together with the *flexor digitorum profundus*[9], this muscle often shows fatigue and stress in musicians. Exercises that prepare this muscle for playing and aid in recovery are *14-Fist out* (page 40) and *15-Fist in* (page 41) along with flexibility exercise *12-Full arm rotations* (page 38).

## 8   Flexor carpi ulnaris

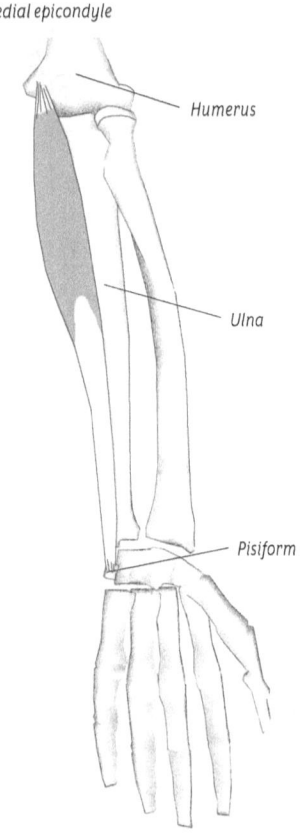

*Medial epicondyle*
*Humerus*
*Ulna*
*Pisiform*

**Location:** The flexor carpi ulnaris has its origin in the medial epicondyle of the humerus and in the posterior border of the ulna. It ends in the carpus, in the pisiform bone, and the base of the fifth metacarpal bone.

**Function:** It allows for the *flexion of the wrist* and *ulnar deviation* (tilting of the hand toward the little finger). It also aids in the *flexion of the elbow*.

**Example:** This muscle is engaged when the wrist is tilted toward the little finger and is commonly used by string musicians. As the right hand moves the bow over the strings from the tip to the frog, it moves from an *extension of the wrist* and *radial deviation* to a *flexion of the wrist* and *ulnar deviation*. It is in this latter movement when the flexor carpi ulnaris comes into play. When pianists stretch their hand to play a ninth, intending to *extend* the little finger as far as possible, their wrist inclines towards this finger by contracting the flexor carpi ulnaris.

**Exercise:** For musicians who wish to make this muscle more flexible or toned, it is helpful to do exercises *12-Full arm rotations* (page 38) and *11-Ping-pong balls* (page 37). To relax and offset stress, see stretch *18-Hand inclined* (page 43).

## 9   Flexor digitorum profundus

**Location:** The flexor digitorum profundus extends from the front of the ulna and the interosseous membrane to the base of the third phalanx of each finger (except the thumb).

**Function:** This muscle bends the third phalanx onto the second and participates in the *flexion* of the phalanges.

**Example:** The flexor digitorum profundus is used when pressing a key on the piano, covering a tone hole on the flute, pushing a piston on the trumpet, or using the left hand on the fretboard of a guitar. A double bass player also uses this muscle when holding a bow.

**Exercise:** For obvious reasons, this muscle is used by most instrumentalists and works similarly to the *extensor digitorum communis*[7]. It is also used in daily activities, which makes it prone to becoming overstressed. This stress can be relieved by stretching with exercises *16-Hand back* (page 42), *17-Hand down* (page 42), or *3-Hand muscles* (page 31). Increase flexibility with *2-Finger mobility 2* (page 30) and strength with exercise *11-Ping-pong balls* (page 37).

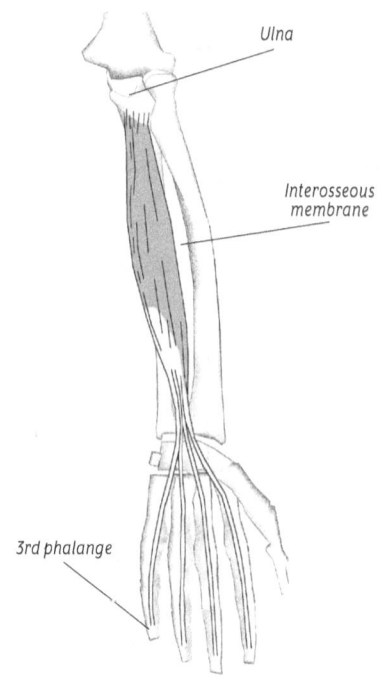

## 10 Gluteus maximus

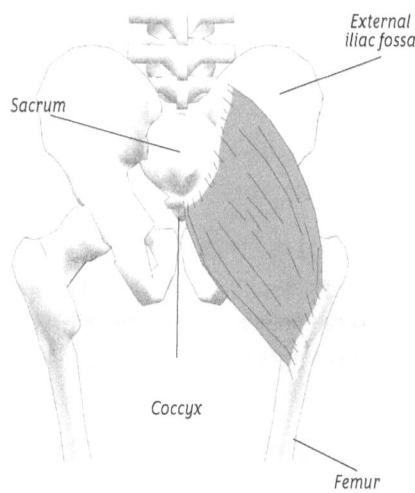

**Location:** The gluteus maximus originates in the sacrum, the coccyx, and the external iliac fossa. It is inserted in the linea aspera of the femur.

**Function:** This muscle enables the *extension* and the external rotation of the leg. When acting in conjunction with the muscle on the opposing side, it bends the pelvis backwards (straightens the lumbar curve).

**Exercise:** Due to the fact that it is not an essential muscle for musicians, it is suggested to be stretched only in a general maintenance program with *54-Glutes* (page 75).

## 11  Hamstring muscles

This muscle set is formed by three muscles called semimembranosus, semitendinosus, and biceps femoris.

**Location:** The three muscles originate in the ischium and descend behind the thigh, inserting in the proximal part of the leg.

**Function:** The semimembranosus and the semitendinosus are involved in the internal rotation and *flexion of the knee*. They also *extend* and help the internal rotation of the hip.

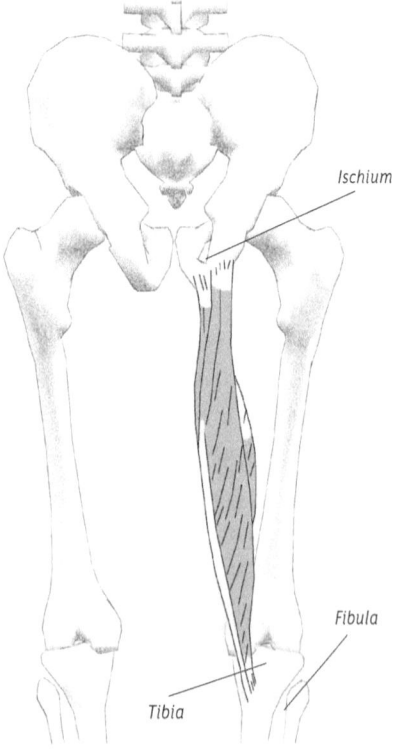

The biceps femoris is responsible for the *flexion* and external rotation of the knee joint, and the *extension* of the hip.

If the lower limb is fixed (i.e., resting on the ground), these muscles shift the pelvis backward (reducing the lumbar curve).

**Example:** When a musician is seated, the hamstrings are contracted (shortened) and the back muscles are relaxed. This tends to cause the musician to lose lumbar curvature, which is clearly harmful for vertebral health.

**Exercise:** All musicians, whether they play seated or standing, must stabilize their pelvis to maintain proper lumbar curvature. Since this involves a muscle group that tends to shrink, it is recommended, mainly to promote better posture when playing, to stretch this muscle group with exercises *52-Leg back 1* (page 73) and *53-Leg back 2* (page 74).

## 12 Iliopsoas

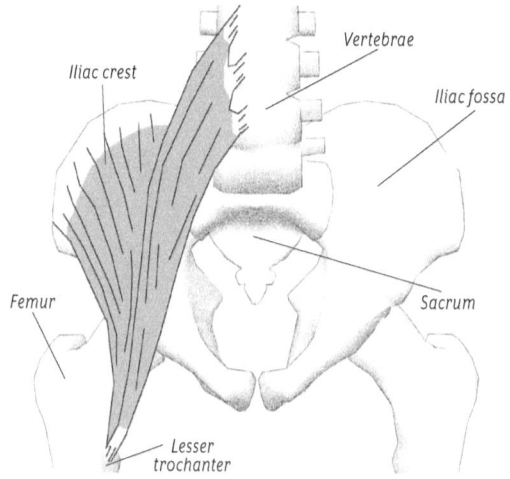

**Location:** The iliopsoas is formed by two muscles: the psoas major muscle and the iliacus muscle. The psoas major goes from the lumbar vertebrae and the last thoracic vertebrae to the lesser trochanter of the femur. The iliacus originates at the iliac cavity, the iliac crest, and the base of the sacrum and travels to the femur.

**Function:** Principally, it controls the *flexion* of the thigh. When the iliopsoas is fixed at the insertion point (i.e., standing up) and both sides on the body are activated, the lumbar curvature (*lordosis*) can be increased.

**Example:** When drummers wish to raise their foot in order to press the bass pedal, the iliopsoas is responsible. If banjo players are seated while playing and feel undue stress on their shoulders caused by leaning their torsos over the instrument, the iliopsoas is used to straighten the back and regain the proper lumbar curvature.

**Exercise:** The iliopsoas along with the *hamstrings*[11] are muscles that tend to contract over years of playing. This has an adverse effect on posture. It is important to prevent the retraction or the shortening of these muscles by means of stretches such as *47-Front hip area* (page 69).

## 13 Latissimus dorsi ("lats")

**Location:** The latissimus dorsi extends from the 7th dorsal vertebra (D7) to the 5th lumbar vertebra (L5). It also connects to the iliac crest as well as the last four ribs and is inserted into the humerus.

**Function:** The latissimus dorsi has various functions. It performs the *internal rotation*, the *adduction* (bringing the elbow closer to the body), and the retropulsion (moving the elbow backward) of the arm. This muscle aids in the hyperextension of the vertebral column (backward inclination of the torso) and can be an accessory muscle for respiration.

# IN TUNE

**Example:** The lats are used by accordion or bagpipe players when deflating the bellows and by percussionists when playing the bongos or the conga drums. For players of instruments such as the guitar, mandolin, lute, ukulele, or banjo, the lats help limit torso rotation, in turn keeping the player's arm from resting on the instrument. For musicians who play large instruments such as the tuba, euphonium, or sousaphone, and even the trumpet, flugelhorn, or bugle, this muscle acts in the same way to keep the instrument and the vertebral column in a suitable playing position.

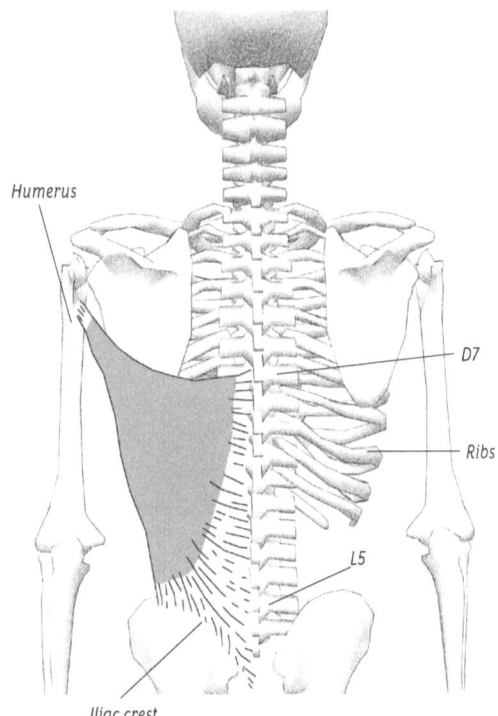

**Exercise:** Since the lats are powerful and strong, musicians must try to maximize their efficacy in order to blow air and play with proper stabilization in the spine and shoulders. The lats are among those muscles that can offset imbalances caused by other muscles such as the *medial deltoid*[16] and muscles near the shoulder, so it is important for musicians to incorporate stretching them in their workout routine with exercise *23-Latissimus dorsi* (page 49) and strengthening them with toning exercises *25-Pillow* (page 50), *26-Chair* (page 51), *27-Pole back* (page 52), *28-Back to the wall* (page 53), and *30-Back with elastic bands* (page 54).

## 14  Levator labii superioris

**Location:** The levator labii superioris goes from the lower border of the orbital bone to the muscles of the upper lip.

**Function:** The levator labii superioris raises and moves the upper lip so as to show the gums.

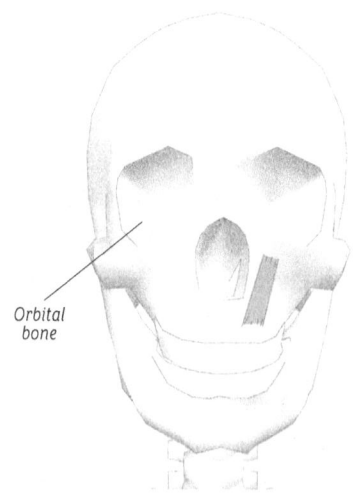

Orbital bone

**Example:** As with the rest of the muscles in the mouth area, primarily due to the fact that all of them are interconnected, the levator labii superioris is used by wind instrument players. The most specific gesture of this muscle is that of puckering the lips while showing the teeth (similar to the mouth of a fish).

**Exercise:** To make this and other muscles of the mouth more flexible, it is worthwhile to do the exercise *59-Vowels and consonants* (page 79). *65-Fish* (page 83) is useful for toning and maintenance of this area.

## 15 Lumbricals of the hand

**Location:** The four lumbricals extend from the tendons of the *flexor digitorum profundus*[9] to the tendons of the *extensor digitorum communis*[7].

**Function:** They perform the same actions as the *palmar interossei muscles*[19].

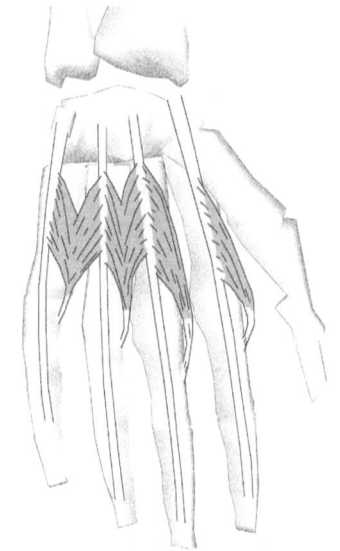

**Exercise:** If the lumbricals are not properly used, the position in which the hand is held can be detrimental to the knuckles (excessive *extension* of the *metacarpophalangeal joints*). This can be observed in the left hand of a guitar player when the movement is generated from the *metacarpophalangeal joints* instead of the *interphalangeal joints*. This is also seen when a pianist excessively flattens the hand and loses the vault shape of the palm. To avoid this, the lumbricals should be toned with exercises *8-Intrinsic plus* (page 34) and *7-Picking up marbles* (page 34), and stretched with *3-Hand muscles* (page 31).

## 16 Medial deltoid

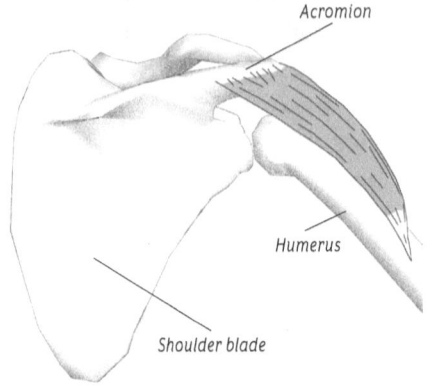

**Location:** The medial deltoid originates from the outer border of the acromion and inserts into the external upper arm, on the outer part of the humerus, at the deltoid tuberosity along with the other two heads of the deltoids (*anterior*[2] and *posterior deltoid*[22]).

**Function:** The medial deltoid performs the *abduction* of the shoulder joint (raising the arms creating a cross or "T" shape).

**Example:** When harpist raise their elbows or bagpipe players lift their arms to inflate the bellows, they do so thanks to this muscle.

**Exercise:** This muscle is engaged whenever the arms are opened. Therefore, the medial deltoid is heavily utilized when playing an instrument as well as in daily life. This continuous use makes it a powerful muscle that tends to pull outwardly on the shoulder joint. The result is that the tendons in the area become pinched. In order to offset the imbalance, the toning exercises *25-Pillow* (page 50), *26-Chair* (page 51), *27-Pole back* (page 52), *28-Back to the wall* (page 53), *29-Pectoral to the wall* (page 53), *30-Back with elastic band* (page 54), and *31-Pectoral elastic band* (page 55) are recommended.

## 17 Obliques

**Location:** Two muscles make up the obliques: obliquus externus abdominis and obliquus internus abdominis. They extend from the lower borders of the last eight ribs to the iliac crest and are interwoven with the opposing muscle, forming the linea alba. This extends from the xiphoid process to the pubis symphysis.

**Function:** The oblique muscles are used to rotate and incline the torso. They participate in the proper positioning of the pelvis and the vertebral column. The obliques assist breathing by helping to compress the abdominal and chest cavities.

# APPENDIX A                                              GLOSSARY OF MUSCLES

**Example:** When wind musicians or singers compress their abdominal walls to improve exhalation, they are utilizing the oblique muscles. If vibraphone players wish to play the upper or lower register, they must incline forward and rotate the torso slightly. This movement is controlled by the obliques.

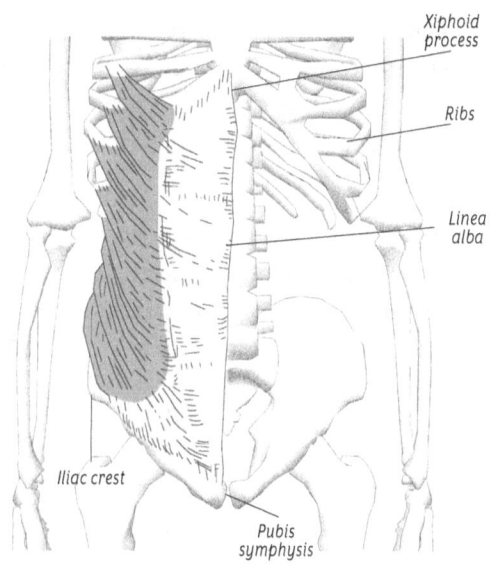

**Exercise:** Breathing properly from the diaphragm is crucial for all wind musicians. It provides for a better sound quality with less fatigue and muscular overload. As indicated by its name, this breathing technique uses the diaphragm and the abdominal muscles in a coordinated manner. Maintaining these muscles in the optimum shape by means of toning exercises *49-Oblique abdominals* (page 70), *50-Abdominal workout using a wall* (page 71), *48-Rectus abdominals* (page 70), and *51-Hamstrings and abdominals* (page 72) provides good posture and better breathing.

## 18  Orbicularis oris

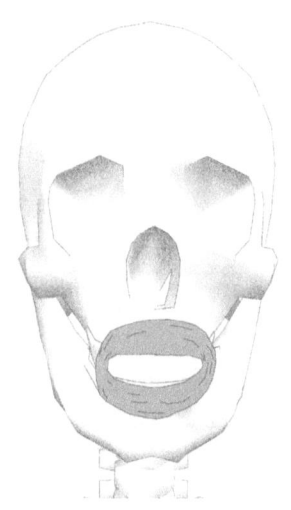

**Location:** The orbicularis oris is located around the opening of the mouth, interconnecting with a network of facial muscles.

**Function:** This muscle allows the lips to purse. However, wind musicians need more than a simple pursing of the lips to play; therefore, the orbicularis muscle combines action with other muscles in order to create the proper structure and form. This is accomplished by simultaneous contraction of the orbicularis oris and the muscles (*caninus*[4], *zygomaticus major*[37], *depressor labii inferiosis*[5], *levator labii superioris*[14], or *risorius*[28], etc.) interconnected with it.

# IN TUNE

**Example:** When trumpet players wish to reach high notes, they must increase the compression of the air stream and engagement of the corners of the lips so that, when the air passes through the lips, a higher vibrational frequency occurs. This engagement is achieved by increasing the contraction of the orbicularis muscle through the control of the muscles surrounding it.

**Exercise:** Wind musicians are generally more aware of the need to warm up in order to condition their lips. Consequently, in addition to the warm-up routine played on the instrument, the exercise *59-Vowels and consonants* (page 79) can be worthwhile along with stretches *60-One-sided face stretch* (page 80) and *61-Two-sided face stretch* (page 81). The orbicularis oris can be toned with *64-Kiss* (page 83).

## 19   Palmar interossei

**Location:** The three palmar interossei muscles extend from the second, fourth, and fifth metacarpal bones to the base of the first phalange of the same fingers and to the flexor tendons.

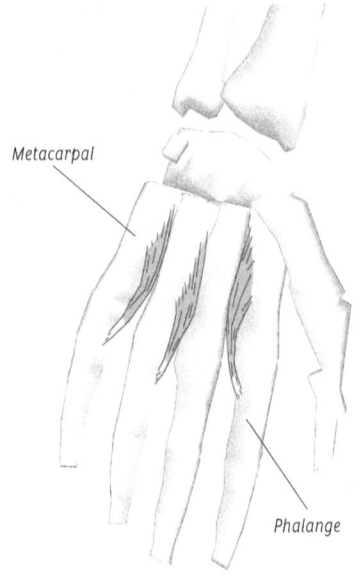
*Metacarpal*

*Phalange*

**Function:** The palmar interossei muscles bring the thumb, index, ring, and little finger close to the middle finger. They also help flex the same fingers with the *extension* of the *proximal* and *distal interphalangeal joints*.

**Example:** In instruments such as the flabiol, txistu, and harmonica, the fingers are generally completely stretched out when playing, and are *flexed* only near the *metacarpophangeal joint*. This is achieved by the action of the palmar interossei together with the *lumbricals of the hand*[15]. Similarly, when playing some notes on the guitar or violin, the little finger on the left hand fully *extends* the *interphalangeal joint* pressing on the string by means of *flexion* of the *metacarpophalangeal joint*.

**Exercise:** The flexibility of *palmar interossei*[19] muscles can be worked with exercise *1-Finger mobility 1* (page 29) and stretched with exercise *3-Hand muscles* (page 31). If these or any of the other intrinsic hand muscles (*dorsal interossei*[6], *palmar interos-*

sei[19], and *lumbricals of the hand*[15]) are weak, the forearm muscles tend to work harder. To avoid this, strengthen the intrinsic hand muscles with *7-Picking up marbles* (page 34) and *8-Intrinsic plus* (page 34).

## 20 Paravertebral muscles

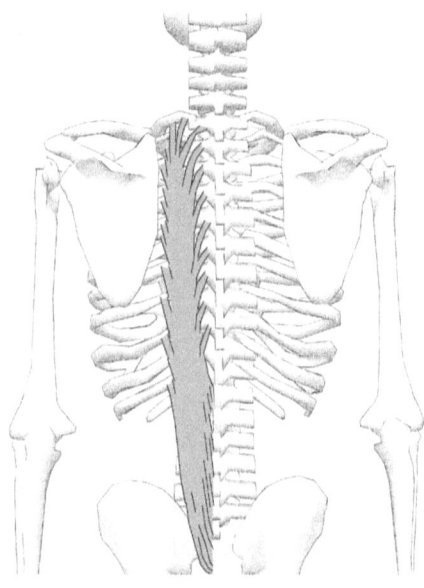

**Location:** The paravertebral muscles go from vertebra to vertebra along the spinal column and are organized into different muscular groups.

**Function:** These muscles are responsible for maintaining the *extension* of the spinal column and the harmonious alignment of the vertebrae.

**Example:** The paravertebral muscles are triggered when adopting or maintaining a straight back, preventing the spinal column from collapsing forward. After a double bass player leans over their instrument to play in the upper register, they resume an erect position thanks to the paravertebral muscles.

**Exercise:** More or less, all instruments and musical activity cause imbalances in the spinal column. This is more noticeable in instruments that require legs and arms to be used simultaneously (drums, organs, harps, etc.). Since the paravertebral muscles are involved in maintaining body equilibrium, it is useful to do flexibility and stretching exercises such as *35-Back of the neck* (page 59), *40-Flexing the lumbar spine* (page 64), *41-Child's pose* (page 65), *42-Straightening the lumbar curve on the ground* (page 66), *43-Back* (page 66), and *45-Lower back* (page 68).

## 21 Pectoral muscle

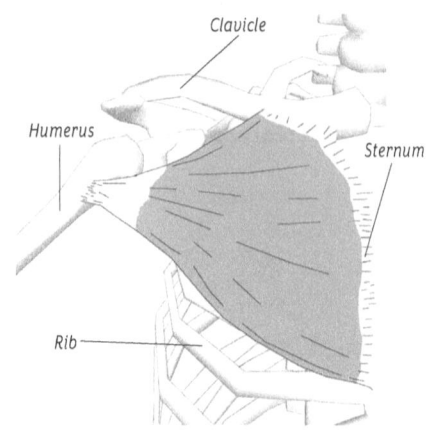

**Location:** The pectoral muscle originates in the sternum, the first ribs, and the clavicle and runs to the upper part of the humerus.

**Function:** This muscle performs *adduction of the arms* (bringing the arms closer to the body) and *internal rotation*.

**Example:** The pectoral muscles come into play when musician's instruments are held in front of them. These muscles are particularly active if effort is exerted on the instrument by bringing the hands or arms together as in the case of the accordion, the concertina, or crash cymbals.

**Exercise:** The shortening of this muscle causes *internal rotation* and *adduction* of the humerus, resulting in the shoulder blade being brought forward and, in turn, separating it from the spinal column and *closing the shoulders*. This position is common in wind musicians. Work on flexibility with exercise *12-Full arm rotations* (page 38) and stretching with exercise *21-Chest* (page 47). If this muscle is weak, the tendons may be pinched from within due to imbalance. If this is the case, do exercises *25-Pillow* (page 50), *26-Chair* (page 51), *29-Pectoral to the wall* (page 53), and *31-Pectoral elastic band* (page 55) to strengthen while avoiding pain and pinched tendons.

## 22 Posterior deltoid

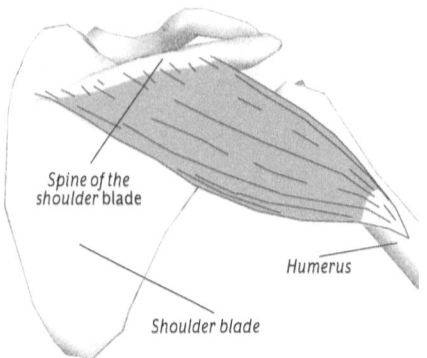

**Location:** The posterior deltoid originates in the spine of the shoulder blade and inserts into the external upper arm, on the outer part of the humerus, at the deltoid tuberosity along with the other two heads of the deltoids (*anterior*[2] and *medial deltoids*[16]).

**Function:** The posterior deltoid performs the extension of the shoulder joint (moves the arm backwards) and contributes to the *external rotation of the arm*.

**Example:** Baritone saxophone players and bassoonists bring the right arm backward when placing their hand on the instrument by means of this muscle. The posterior deltoid also comes into play when a flute player put their hands on the instrument by pulling the right arm back in *external rotation*. It should also be noted that French horn players who hold their bell off the leg utilize this muscle.

**Exercise:** All musicians who bring their arm back, especially those who play larger instruments which are held to the side, can relieve the stress of the posterior deltoid by means of the stretching exercise *24-Rear shoulder* (page 50).

## 23 Quadratus lumborum

**Location:** The quadratus lumborum originates in the Iliac crest and ends in the lower border of the last rib. It is also inserted in the transverse process of the first four lumbar vertebrae through small tendons.

**Function:** This muscle produces the lateral inclination of the vertebral column. It also acts when breathing by lowering the last rib. If contracted with the rest of the back and abdominal muscles, it helps to stabilize the area and maintain good posture.

**Example:** When pianists laterally tilt their spinal column to move their body to better reach the upper part of the keyboard, the quadratus lumborum muscle is being used.

**Exercise:** Because of the quadratus lumborum's effect on the posture of the vertebral column, it is valuable for all musicians to stretch this muscle. It is particularly worthwhile for certain musicians such as drummers or organists, who lack stable support on the ground, to exercise the muscles of this area. Since the quadratus lumborum is used to balance a person's weight, stretching it is also beneficial for

**IN TUNE**

musicians who tend hunch over large instruments, e.g., the djembe drum, double bass, and bassoon.

Wind musicians who must use their diaphragm a good deal, as well as any musicians who must play their instruments for long periods of time, can benefit from exercise *45-Lower back* (page 68), which specifically works this muscle.

## 24 Quadriceps

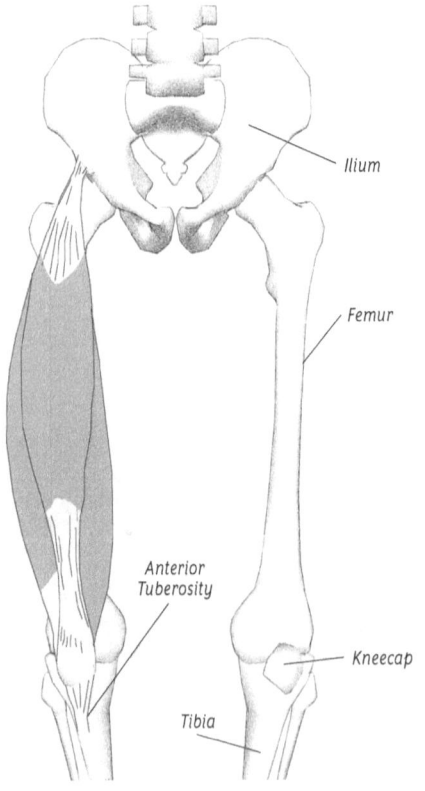

This muscle is one of the most powerful in the body and is comprised of four muscular sets: the rectus femoris, the vastus intermedius, the vastus medialis, and the vastus lateralis.

**Location:** It extends from the ilium and the femur to form a common tendon that passes in front of and is partly inserted into the kneecap. The quadriceps then form part of the patellar tendon (kneecap) and ends in the front of the tibia.

**Function:** This muscle as a whole creates the *extension of the knee*, and a portion of the rectus femoris allows *flexion of the hip*.

**Example:** The quadriceps come into play when an organist takes their foot off the foot rest to search for a pedal or when harpists changes pedal positions.

**Exercise:** Since the quadricep is a powerful muscle, musicians would have difficulty overstressing it regardless of the intensity of the activity. Accordingly, it is not crucial to include quadricep stretches in the exercise routine. However, since this muscle is also important for most sports activities, daily living, and maintaining good posture, it is wise to stretch it with exercise *57- Front leg* (page 77) in a general fitness regimen.

## 25 Radial muscles

**Location:** These muscle groups are formed by the extensor carpi radialis longus and extensor carpi radialis brevis muscles. The radials travel from the epicondyle of the humerus to the base of the second and third metacarpal bones.

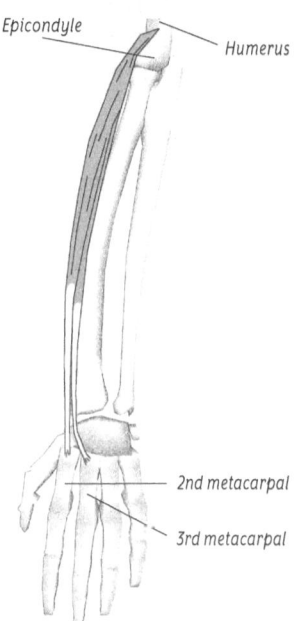

**Function:** The radials perform the *extension of the wrist* with inclination or *radial deviation*.

**Example:** When pianists cross the index finger over the thumb, an *extension* and slight *radial deviation* occur by means of these muscles.

**Exercise:** These muscles often act in conjunction with the *extensor digitorum communis*[7]. As such, they are easily overstressed when practicing. Conditioning the radials using the stretch *13-Wrist down* (page 39) prevents problems in the area.

## 26 Rectus abdominis

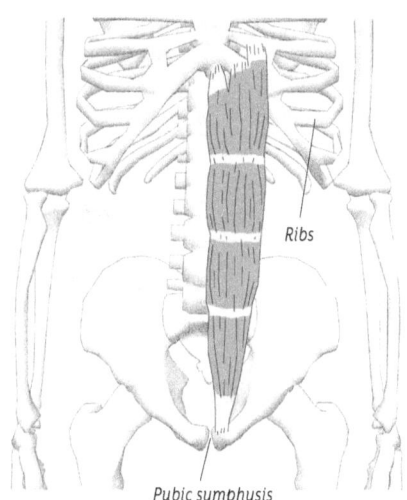

**Location:** The rectus abdominis originates in the cartilage of the fifth, sixth, and seventh ribs and inserts into the pubic symphysis.

**Function:** The basic functions of the rectus abdominis is to create *flexion of the torso* and inhibit the lumbar region from having excessive curvature *(hyperlordosis)*. It also supports and prevents the protrusion of the abdominal wall and contributes to diaphragmatic breathing.

**Example:** When wind musicians need an increase in air pressure to reach the higher notes, their abdominal muscles activate. When an organist or drummer wishes to ensure torso and abdominal stability to better control the arms and legs simultaneously, the back muscles (*paravertebrals*[20], *quadratus lumborum*[23], etc.) and the abdominal muscles synchronically contract.

**Exercise:** All abdominal muscles in general tend to relax and are rarely overstressed. For this reason, it is important to tone them and not necessary to stretch them.

All musicians, wind players in particular, should ensure these muscles are in good shape in order to prevent abdominal distension as well as to avoid an increase in lumbar curvature and tension in the vertebral column. Helpful toning exercises are *48-Rectus abdominals* (page 70), *49-Oblique abdominals* (page 70), *50-Abdominal workout using a wall* (page 71), and *51-Hamstrings and abdominals* (page 72).

## 27 Rhomboid muscles

**Location:** These muscles originate in the sixth cervical vertebra (rhomboid minor) and the first four thoracic vertebra (rhomboid major), ending at the inside border of the shoulder blade.

**Function:** The rhomboid muscles retract (*adduction*), lift, and *internally rotate* the shoulder blade.

**Example:** To more efficiently hold the flute, the right shoulder blade of the flutist moves down and back due to the contraction of the rhomboid muscles. This brings the shoulder blade backward, in turn, stabilizing the shoulder, balancing the spinal column, and improving the freedom of movement in the hand.

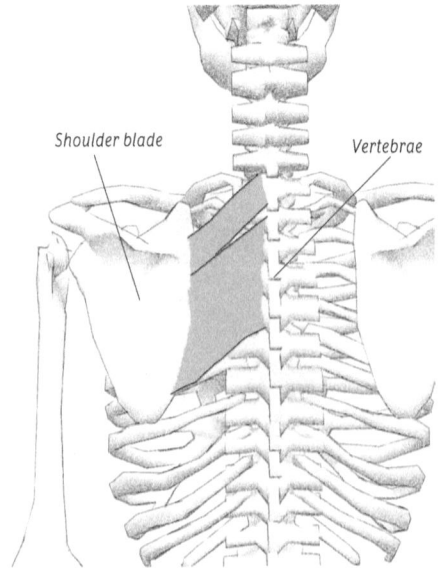

Shoulder blade · Vertebrae

**Exercise:** These muscles are crucial for stabilizing the shoulder blade. The rhomboid muscles of all musicians are subject to significant stress, primarily in those who support their instruments (particularly the heavier instruments, such as the bassoon, baritone saxophone, tenor saxophone, trombone, tuba, euphonium, etc.). Musicians can compensate for these stresses with flexibility exercise *12-Full arm rotations* (page 38) and stretching exercise *39-Interscapular* (page 62).

## 28  Risorius

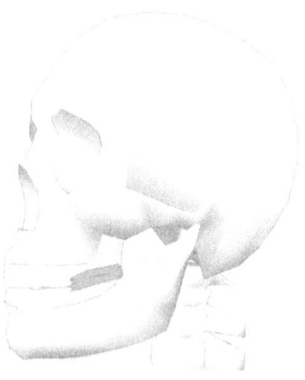

**Location:** This muscle goes from the masseter muscle (not shown in the figure) to the corner of the mouth.

**Function:** The risorius moves the corners of the mouth backward.

**Example:** This muscle is used by every wind instrumentalists because the muscles of the face are all interconnected. The most specific gesture made by this muscle is to pull back the corners of the lips.

**Exercise:** To help keep this muscle flexible, use exercise *59-Vowels and consonants* (page 79). Exercise *62-Straight smile* (page 81) can be used for strengthening purposes.

## 29  Scapula levator

**Location:** The scapula levator runs from the transverse process of the first three cervical vertebrae to the upper medial edge of the shoulder blade.

**Function:** It elevates the shoulder blade as well as participates in its *external rotation* and stabilization. If both scapula levator muscles are simultaneously contracted, they contribute to the *extension of the neck*.

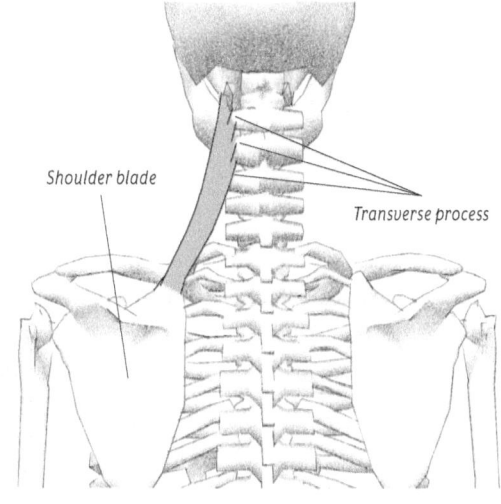

*Shoulder blade*

*Transverse process*

**Example:** This is one of the muscles that makes it possible to grasp the violin or viola between the chin and the shoulder.

**Exercise:** In order to achieve greater interpretive precision, all musicians must stabilize their neck and shoulder blades. Therefore, the scapula levator tends to be worked with an excessive amount of tension. In addition, muscular tension of the area is increased by technically difficult music, mental stress, and even cold temperatures. Exercises that assist in relaxing this region are *19-Raising and lowering the shoulders* (page 46), *35-Back of the neck* (page 59), and *38-Scapula levator* (page 61).

## 30 Short extensor of the thumb

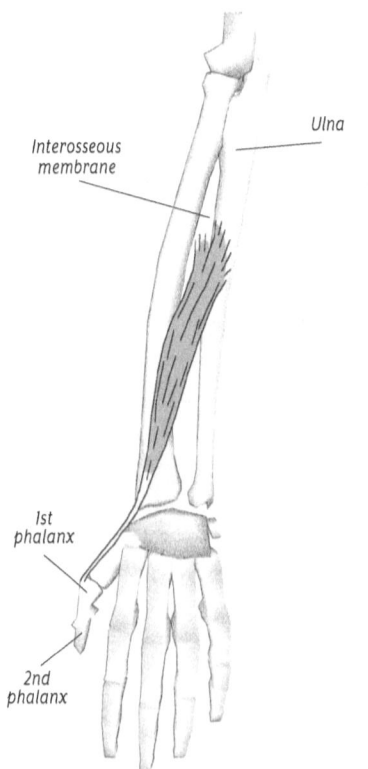

**Location:** The short extensor of the thumb goes from the posterior aspect of the ulna and the interosseous membrane to the dorsal aspect of the first phalanx of the thumb.

**Function:** This muscle performs the *extension* of the *metacarpophalangeal joint*. The thumb also has another extensor muscle known as the long extensor, which is inserted into the second phalanx. Unlike the short extensor, the long extensor of the thumb enables the entire finger to *extend*.

**Example:** When guitarists play an ascending arpeggio, the right hand begins with the thumb and may be followed by the index, middle, and ring fingers. After the thumb has already plucked the string, the extensor muscle is used to return it to the initial position. Additionally, oboists support the weight of the oboe in the right hand using this muscle, unless a neck strap is used.

**Exercise:** To make this muscle more flexible, exercises *1-Finger mobility 1* (page 29) and *2-Finger mobility 2* (page 30) can be used. For stretching, perform exercise *5-Thumb down* (page 32) and for toning perform exercises *9-Rubber bands* (page 35) and *11-Ping-pong balls* (page 37).

## 31  Short flexor of the thumb

**Location:** The short flexor of the thumb originates in the front part of the carpus (wrist) and extends to the base of the first phalanx of the thumb.

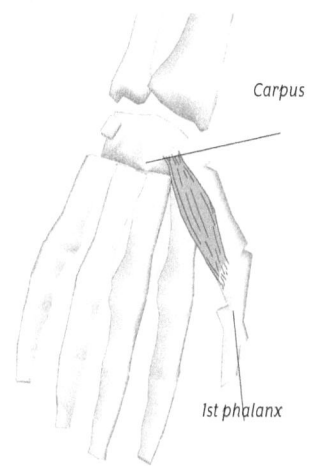

**Function:** This muscle *flexes the thumb* and pulls it forward (towards the palm).

**Example:** This muscle is utilized when pressing the octave key on a woodwind instrument such as the clarinet, saxophone, bassoon, flute, or oboe. The short flexor of the thumb is also brought into play when any string musician presses on the back of the neck of the instrument with the thumb.

**Exercise:** As with all hand muscles, this is a small muscle. Accordingly, it can easily fail if it is overstressed or not given enough time to relax. To improve flexibility, use exercise *2-Finger mobility 2* (page 30) and to stretch it use *6-Thumb back* (page 33) or *4-Palm of the hand* (page 31).

## 32  Splenius

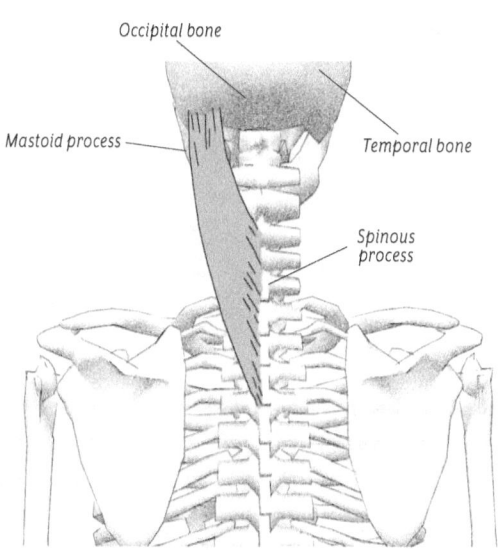

**Location:** The splenius muscle originates in the spinous process of the last cervical and first thoracic vertebrae and ends in the mastoid process of the temporal bone and the occipital bone.

**Function:** If both sides of splenius muscles are activated, this causes the *extension of the head*. If only one side is stimulated, this produces a lateral inclination and rotation to that side.

# IN TUNE

**Example:** When trumpet players raise the bell of the instrument, both splenius muscles are contracted simultaneously. When violinists place the instrument between the chin and shoulder, the splenius on the left side is used.

**Exercise:** One of the most important concepts for obtaining and maintaining a good posture is pursuing verticality of the body. In regard to the cervical spine, the splenius is one of the primary muscles used to obtain this verticality. As with the other cervical and thoracic muscles, the splenius tends to accumulate tension and become contracted. Promote mobility by doing flexibility exercises *32-Yes with the neck* (page 57), *33-Maybe with the neck* (page 58), and *34-No with the neck* (page 59) as well as stretches *35-Back of the neck* (page 59) and *43-Back* (page 66).

## 33  Sternocleidomastoid

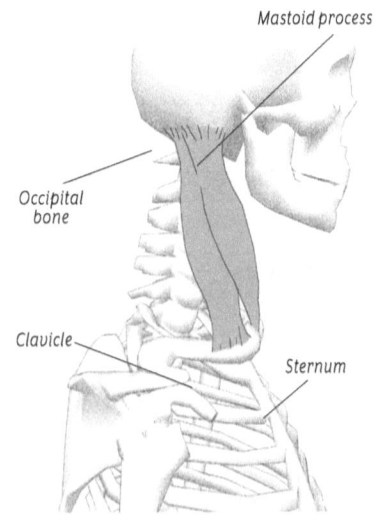

**Location:** The sternocleidomastoid extends from the sternum and the clavicle to the mastoid process and the occipital bone.

**Function:** The sternocleidomastoid muscle produces the lateral inclination toward the side of the contraction and the *extension* and *rotation* of the opposite side. If the muscles on both sides are simultaneously activated, they produce an *extension of the head*, accentuating the cervical *lordosis*. When both sides are contracted along with other muscles of the cervical area, the neck is powerfully stabilized.

**Example:** The contraction of the sternocleidomastoid of guitar players enables them to move their head so that they can watch where they are placing the fingers of the left hand on the strings.

**Exercise:** As with the rest of the muscles in the area, this muscle has a significant tendency to become overstressed. Therefore, all musicians should cultivate flexibility by performing *32-Yes with the neck* (page 57), *33-Maybe with the neck* (page 58), and *34-No with the neck* (page 59) as well as doing stretching exercises *36-Front of the neck* (page 60), *35-Back of the neck* (page 59), and *43-Back* (page 66).

# APPENDIX A　　　　　　　　　　　　　　　　　　　　　GLOSSARY OF MUSCLES

## 34 Trapezius

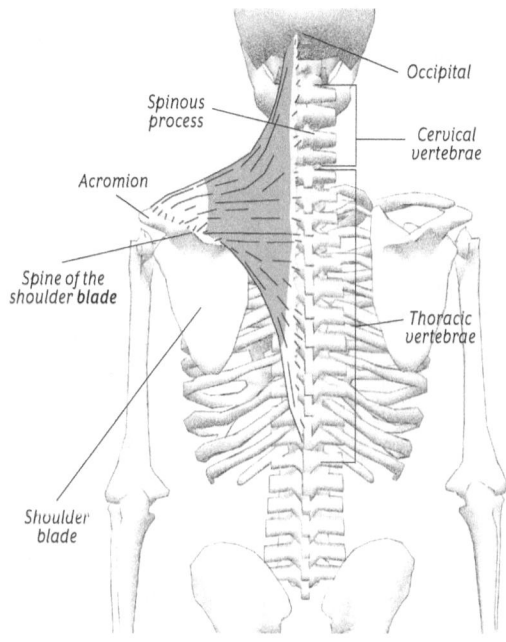

**Location:** The trapezius muscle originates in the occipital and the spinous process of all of the cervical vertebrae and all thoracic vertebrae up to the tenth. The points of insertion are the rear border of the clavicle, the acromion, and the spine of the shoulder blade.

**Function:** The trapezius muscle raises and depresses the shoulder blade by contracting the upper and lower fibers. Accordingly, it is an essential muscle for stabilizing the shoulder blade to the torso. The trapezius muscle is also responsible for the *adduction* of the shoulder.

**Example:** When musicians raise their shoulders, the upper part of the trapezius muscle is used.

**Exercise:** As with the *rhomboid muscles*[27], the trapezius allows for improved freedom of movement in the hands due to the stabilization of the shoulder blade. Subsequently, the trapezius is frequently used by musicians and is prone to excessive tightening. In situations of stress or cold, it tends to tense up easily. Accordingly, it is not unusual to see musicians who have hunched shoulders and even discomfort or pain in this area. Use flexibility exercises *19-Raising and lowering the shoulders* (page 46) and *33-Maybe with the neck* (page 58) and stretching exercises *35-Back of the neck* (page 59), *37-Side of the neck* (page 61), and *38-Scapula levator* (page 61) to work these muscles.

## 35 Triceps brachii

**Location:** This muscle is formed by three parts: the long head originating in the shoulder blade, and the lateral and medial heads beginning in the dorsal part of the humerus. These three heads connect at a common tendon ending in the olecranon.

**Function:** The triceps brachii is responsible for *extending the elbow*.

**Example:** When percussionists strike the marimba, the triceps contract, adding speed and force to the impact.

The triceps contract when violinists stretch their arm to run the bow from the frog to the tip.

**Exercise:** This area can be stretched with exercise *22-Posterior arm muscles* (page 48).

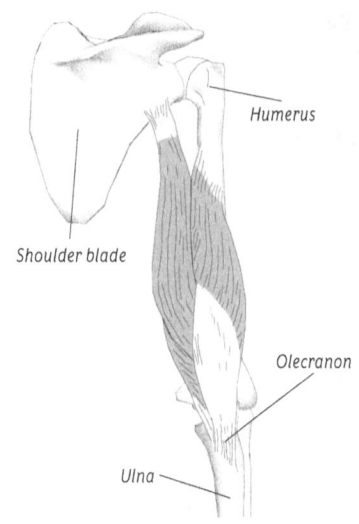

## 36 Triceps surae

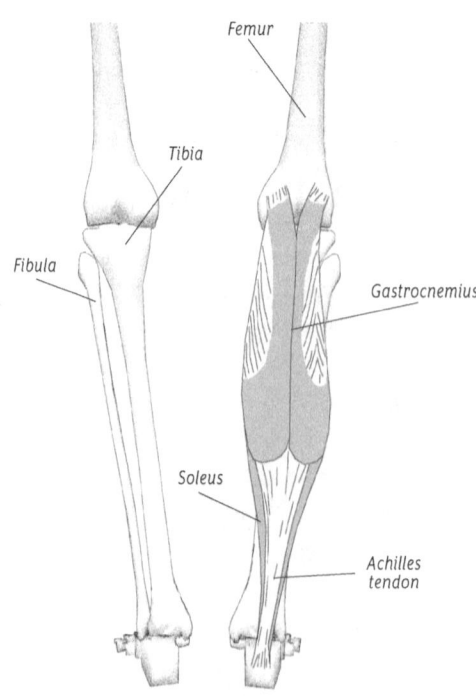

**Location:** This muscle is the strongest leg muscle and is formed by three muscle heads: the soleus and both heads of the gastrocnemius. The soleus originates in the upper dorsal region of the tibia and fibula. The gastrocnemius originates at the base of the femur. They are jointly inserted in the Achilles tendon.

**Function:** The triceps surae induces plantar *flexion* of the ankle (pointing the toes).

**Example:** When organists, percussionists, or harpists press a pedal, this motion is .00 accomplished by both the triceps surae, which points the toes down, and gravity. The triceps surae is also used when marching musicians lift their heel off the ground to take a step.

**Exercise:** Obviously, pointing the toes is not an essential movement for most musicians. However, due to its role in daily life, *58-Calf muscles* (page 78) is a useful exercise within the general conditioning program for musicians.

## 37 Zygomaticus major

**Location:** The zygomaticus major extends from the zygomatic arch (cheekbone) to the corner of the mouth and is interlaced with the adjacent muscles.

**Function:** It draws the corner of the mouth upward and outward.

**Example:** As all the muscles of the mouth area are interconnected, the zygomaticus major is used by all wind musicians. The most specific action of this muscle is smiling.

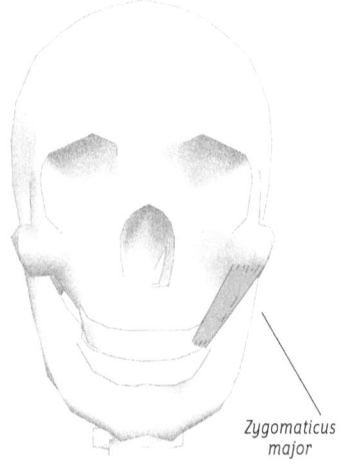

Zygomaticus major

**Exercise:** To make this and the other muscles of the mouth more flexible, exercise *59-Vowels and consonants* (page 79) may be worthwhile. Exercise *67-Upward smile* (page 84) is useful for toning this area.

Appendix

# GLOSSARY OF TERMS

Below are the medical terms cited in the text. They are listed in alphabetical order.

## ABDUCTION OF THE ARM

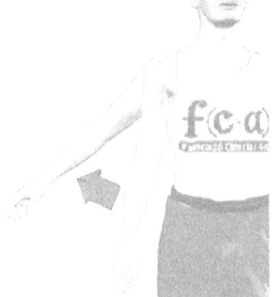

Separating the arm laterally from the body.

## ADDUCTION OF THE ARM

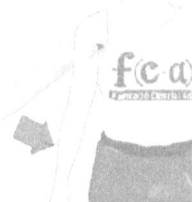

Bringing the arm closer to the body.

## CLOSING THE SHOULDERS

Moving and sustaining the shoulders forward. This creates tension in the musculature of the cervical area, thoracic region, and the shoulders. It also makes proper breathing difficult.

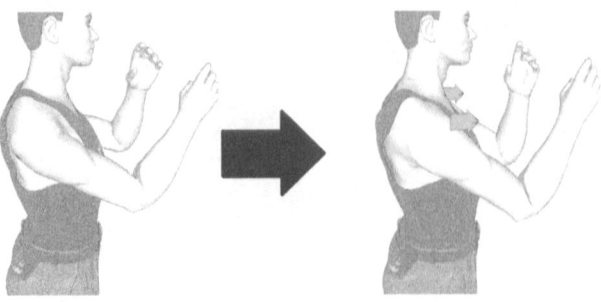

## DISTAL INTERPHALANGEAL JOINTS

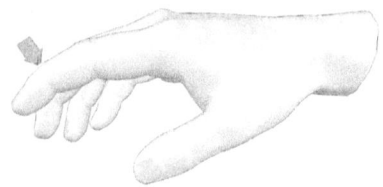

Union between two distal phalanges (2nd and 3rd phalanges).

## DORSAL HUNCHING

Accentuation of the trunk curvature (kyphosis), a combination of thoracic hunching and pelvis rotation.

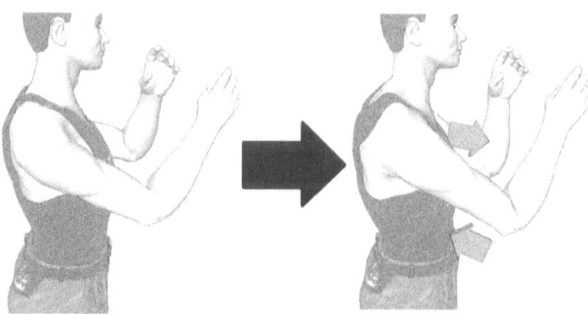

## EXTENSION

A straightening motion.

## EXTENSION OF THE ANKLE

Lifting the top of the foot toward the leg, as when walking on one's heels.

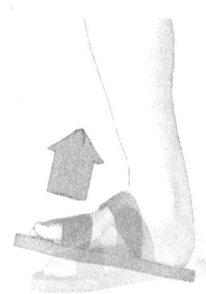

## EXTENSION OF THE ELBOW (STRAIGHTENING)

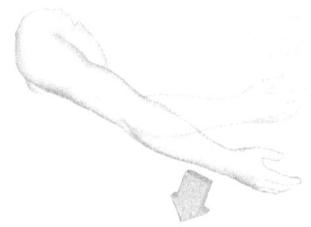

Stretching the arm, placing the elbow in a straight position.

## EXTENSION OF A FINGER

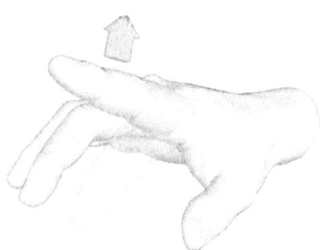

Stretching the various joints of a finger into a straight position.

## EXTENSION OF THE HEAD/NECK

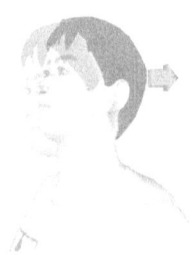

Moving the head backward, tilting the chin upwards.

## EXTENSION OF THE KNEE

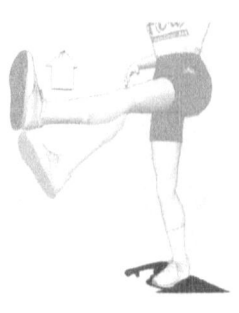

Stretching the leg, lifting it to a straight position.

## EXTENSION OF THE THUMB

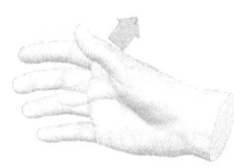

Lifting the thumb backward, stretching the interphalangeal and *metacarpophalangeal joints*.

## EXTENSION OF THE WRISTS

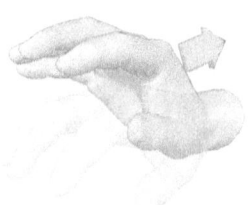

Pulling the hand backward, exposing the palm.

## EXTERNAL ROTATION OF THE ARM OR THE HAND (SUPINATION)

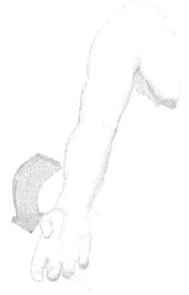

Turning the palm of the hand up by twisting the arm or forearm.

## FLEXION

A bending motion.

## FLEXION OF THE ELBOW (ELBOW BENT)

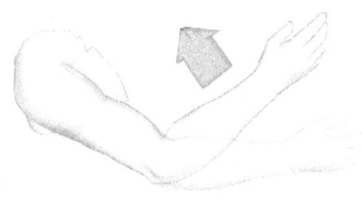

Bending the elbow, bringing the forearm toward the *bicep*.

## FLEXION OF A FINGER

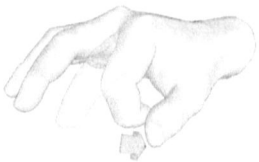

Bringing a finger toward the palm of the hand, bending all of its joints.

## FLEXION OF THE HEAD

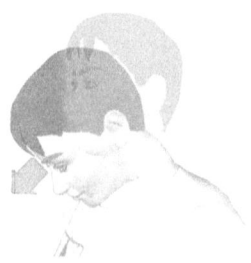

Lowering the head forward, bringing the chin closer to the chest.

## FLEXION OF THE HIP (HIP BENT)

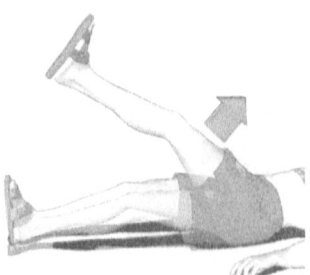

Bending the hip, bringing the thigh closer to the abdomen.

## FLEXION OF THE KNEE (KNEE BENT)

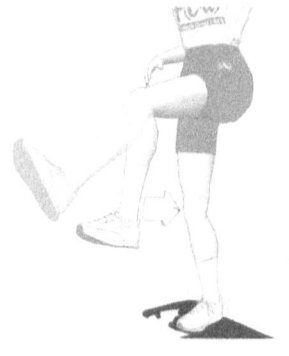

Bending the knee, lifting the foot toward the buttock.

## FLEXION OF THE THUMB

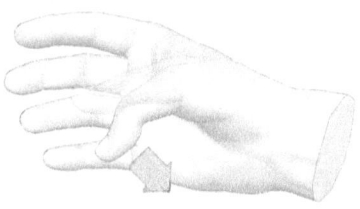

Bending the thumb inside the palm of the hand toward the little finger.

## FLEXION OF THE TORSO

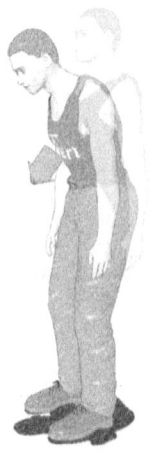

Lowering the chest, tilting the body forward.

## FLEXION OF THE WRIST

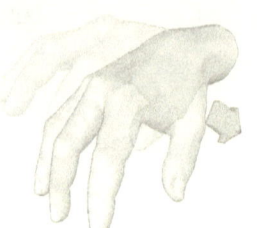

Bending the hand down, bringing the palm of the hand to the inner part of the forearm.

## HYPEREXTENSION DUE TO BEING DOUBLE JOINTED (HYPERMOBILITY)

The increased slackness of the *metacarpophangeal joint* of the thumb allows for excessive *extension*. This movement can potentially harm the joints of the thumb as well as its tendons.

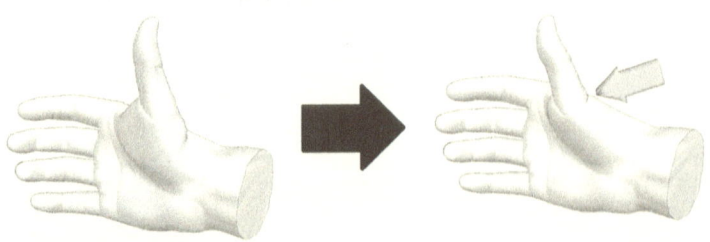

## HYPERLORDOSIS

Over-accentuating the curvature of the spine.

## INCLINATION OF THE HEAD/NECK (TILTING)

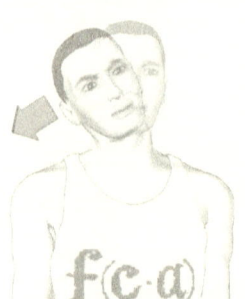

A lateral tilting movement of the head, placing the ear close to the shoulder.

## INTERNAL ROTATION OF THE ARM OR HAND (PRONATION)

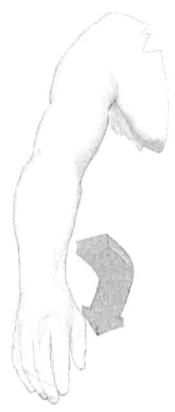

Turning the palm of the hand downward by twisting the arm or forearm.

## LORDOSIS

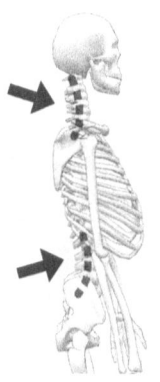

Curve formed by the lumbar and cervical column, showing a posterior concavity.

## METACARPOPHALANGEAL JOINT

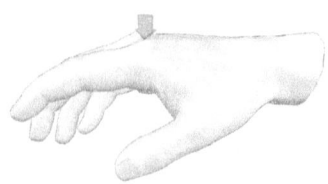

Union between the 1st phalange and the metacarpal bone, at the base of the fingers.

## MUSCLE CONTRACTION (SPASM)

The involuntary and unnecessary activation of a muscle. This results in reduced fluidity of movement. If the muscle tension goes beyond a certain limit, it can be uncomfortable or painful.

## PROXIMAL INTERPHALANGEAL JOINT

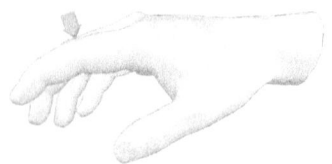

Union between the two phalanges closest to the base of the fingers (1st and 2nd phalanges).

## RADIAL DEVIATION

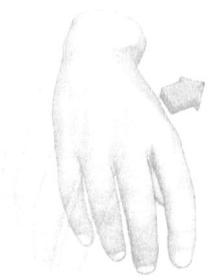

Lateral tilting of the wrist to the side, toward the thumb and the radius.

## ROTATION OF THE HEAD

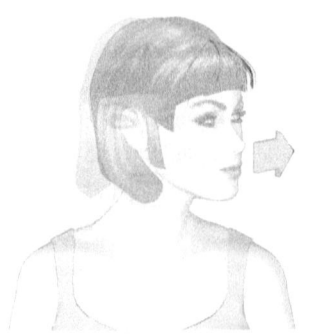

Looking to one side by twisting the neck with the chin tracking over the shoulder.

## STRAIGHTENING THE LUMBAR CURVE (REDUCE LORDOSIS)

A backward movement of the pelvis and the spine that reduces the curvature of the lumbar area.

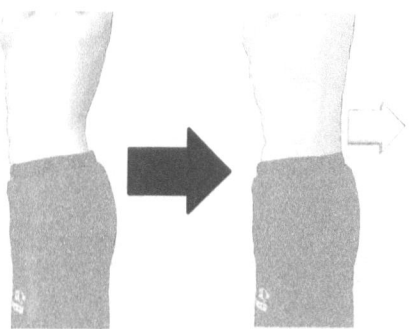

## ULNAR DEVIATION

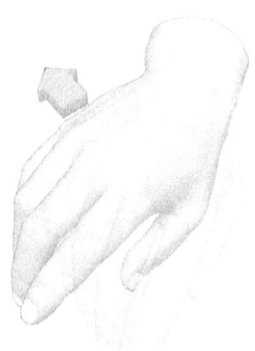

Lateral tilting of the wrist toward the side of the little finger and the ulna.

# Index

| | |
|---|---|
| abdominals | 64-72 |
|     flexibility | 64-66 |
|     hyperextension | 255 |
|     lateral (oblique) | 67, 70, 256, 263, 272-273, 280 |
|     rectus muscle | 70, 278-280 |
|     toning | 64, 70-72 |
|     wall | 71 |
| abduction | 7, 30, 55 |
| Achilles tendon | 78 |
| adduction | 7, 30, 260, 269, 276 |
| adductor muscles | 76-77, 260-261 |
| aerobic | 24, 228 |
| anaerobic | 24 |
| arms | 38-56, 106, 115, 140, 149, 166, 185, 192 |
| back | 49-50, 57-60, 64-72, 140, 157, 166, 192 |
|     flexibility | 51-52, 64-65 |
|     lower, see *lumbar stretching* | 68 |
|     stretching | 66-67 |
|     toning | 75 |
| bicep muscle | 47, 261-262 |
| biceps femori muscle | 268 |
| body awareness | 14 |
| brass | 209-226 |
|     cooling down | 214-217, 223-226 |
|     warming up | 209-214, 218-223 |
| breathing | 16, 64, 250, 272, 273, 277, 279, 290 |
| caninus muscle | 263, 273 |
| cardiorespiratory endurance | 19 |
| cervical, see *neck* | |
| cervical curvature | 64, 74, 253, 254 |
| chest | 45-56 |
| children | 8, 15 |
| cooling down | 24-26, 88-89 |
|     brass | 214-217, 223-226 |
|     harp | 171-174 |
|     keyboard | 197-199, 205-208 |
|     percussion | 180-182, 188-191 |
|     strings | 137-139, 145-148, 154-156, 162-165 |
|     winds | 101-105, 111-113, 119-122, 128-131 |
| cramping | 84 |
| deltoid muscles | 50, 270 |
|     anterior | 261, 272 |
|     medial | 261, 270, 272 |
|     posterior | 270, 272, 276-277 |
| dorsa muscles | 29, 34-35, 264, 269, 282 |
| dorsal region | 29, 57-63 |
| drum set | 183-191 |

| | |
|---|---|
| eating | 15 |
| elastic band | 54-56 |
| elasticity | 4, 7-8, 12-13, 19, 21, 29, 53, 81-84 |
| elbows | 38-43, 48-63, 106, 123, 132, 149, 166, 262 |
| endurance | 19 |
| equipment | 16, 21-22, 74 |
| extension | 9, 32, 42 |
| extensor digitorum communis | |
|     muscle | 29, 39, 40-41, 264-266, 271, 279 |
| extensor carpi radialis muscles | 279 |
| face | 79-85, 211, 218 |
|     flexibility | 79-80 |
|     stretching | 80-81 |
|     toning | 81-85 |
| fingers | 7, 29-37, 125, 192, 264-275 |
|     flexor adaptation | 247 |
|     thumb adaptation | 248 |
| flexibility | 7-12, 16-17, 24-26 |
| flexion | 7, 31, 37, 39, 60 |
| flexor carpi ulnaris | 29, 42-43, 266 |
| flexor digitorum profundus | |
|     muscle | 29, 42, 247, 266-267, 271 |
| flexor muscles | 36, 49 |
| forearm | 38-44, 149, 192 |
|     flexibility | 38-39 |
|     stretching | 39-43 |
|     toning | 44 |
| gastrocnemius muscle | 286 |
| glutes | 75 |
| gluteus maximus muscle | 65, 75, 77, 267 |
| hamstrings | 72, 75-77, 256, 268, 273, 280 |
| hands | 29-46, 132, 140, 166, 175, , 192, 200 |
|     flexibility | 29-30 |
|     hyperextension | 34 |
|     stretching | 31-33 |
|     toning | 34-37 |
|     wrist adaptation | 247 |
| harp | 166-176 |
|     cooling down | 171-176 |
|     warming up | 166-171 |
| head | 57-65, 253-254 |
| hips | 69, 268, 294 |
| hyperextension | 34, 253-254 |
| hyperlordosis | 49-50, 53, 77 |
| hypertrophy | 20 |
| iliopsoas muscle | 69, 269 |
| instrument groups | 90-95 |

301

| | | | |
|---|---|---|---|
| interscapular | 62 | pole | 22, 52 |
| intrinsic muscles | 29-35, 264, 271, 274-275 | posterior arm muscles | 50 |
| irradiation | 77 | posture | 8-9, 20, 22, 47, 57, 59, 60, 64, 66, 68 |
| isometric | 21-23, 38-39, 53 | quadriceps | 77, 260, 278 |
| isotonic | 21-22 | quadratus lumborum | 68, 71, 277, 280 |
| juggling | 36 | radial deviation | 43, 266, 279, 298 |
| keyboard | 192-208 | radial muscles | 29, 39, 50, 279 |
|     cooling down | 197-199, 205-208 | radial tuberosity | 261-262 |
|     warming up | 192-196, 200-205 | range of motion | 7, 17, 22, 29, 45 |
| lactic acid | 14 | rectus abdominis | 70, 256, 275, 279 |
| latissimus dorsi | 49-50, 269-270 | rectus femoris muscle | 278 |
| legs | 73-78 | repetitions | 22 |
|     flexibility | 73 | rhomboid muscles | 62-63, 280-281, 285 |
|     stretching | 73-78 | risorius muscle | 273, 281 |
|     toning | 78 | rubber ball | 36 |
| levator labii superioris muscle | 270-273 | rubber bands | 35 |
| lumbar | 64-72, 76, 218 | sacrum | 66, 70 |
|     flexibility | 64-66 | scapula levator | 61-62, 249, 281-282 |
|     hyperextension | 254 | semimembranosus muscle | 268 |
|     stretching | 66-69 | semitendinosus muscle | 268 |
|     toning | 70-72 | short extensor of the thumb muscle | 32, 265, 282 |
| lumbrical muscles | 29, 31, 34-35, 264, 271, 274-275 | shoulders | 45-56, 96, 106, 114, 123, 132 |
| lymphatic flow | 14 | | 149, 166, 183, 209 |
| marbles | 34 |     flexibility | 45-47, 57, 61-63 |
| masseter muscle | 281 |     stretching | 47-50 |
| metabolic | 24-26 |     toning | 50-56 |
| metacarpophalangeal joint | 31-36, 264 | soleus muscle | 286 |
| mimic muscles | 79 | spine | 72, 132, 158, 183, 192, 200, 218 |
| mirror | 16 |     flexing | 64 |
| musculoskeletal conditioning | 19 |     stretching | 48, 68-69 |
| neck | 13, 57-63, 64, 67, 248-249, 253, 281-285, 298 |     tension | 57-58 |
|     flexibility | 57-59 |     twist adaptation | 250 |
|     hyperextension | 253 | splenius muscle | 62, 59-60, 249, 283-284 |
|     hyperflexion | 253 | sternocleidomastoid muscle | 57, 60, 249, 284 |
|     stretch adaptation | 248-249 | stick | 21, 52 |
|     stretching | 59-63 | strength | 3, 7, 19-21 |
|     toning | 63 | stress | 14, 16-17 |
| nerves | 24, 265 | stretching | 13-21 |
| obliques | 272-273 | string instruments, bowed, front | 132-139 |
| orbicularis oris | 83-85, 275-276 |     cooling down | 137-139 |
| pain | 14-17, 20 |     warming up | 132-136 |
| palmar aponeurosis | 31 | string instruments, bowed, large | 140-148 |
| palmar interossei | 29, 31, 34-37, 264-265, 271, 274 |     cooling down | 145-148 |
| paravertebral muscles | 66, 275, 280 |     warming up | 140-145 |
| pectineus muscle | 260 | string instruments, bowed, shoulder | 149-156 |
| pectoral muscles | 47-48, 53-54, 55-56, 276-277 |     cooling down | 154-156 |
| pelvis | 73-78 |     warming up | 149-153 |
| percussion | 175-191 | string instruments, plucked | 157-165 |
|     cooling down | 180-182, 188-191 |     cooling down | 162-165 |
|     warming up | 175-179, 185-188 |     warming up | 157-162 |
| pillow | 21, 50-51, 74 | temporomandibular | 80 |
| ping-pong balls | 37 | tendons | 7, 13-14, 29, 49, 50, 53, 88 |

# INDEX

| | |
|---|---|
| tension in muscles | 13-17, 19, 22, 25 |
| thighs | 75-78 |
|     flexibility | 75 |
|     stretching | 75-78 |
|     toning | 78 |
| thoracic region | 63, 67, 75, 229, 284 |
| thumb | 13, 14, 31-36, 40-43, 96, 248, 264, 274, 282-283, 293, 295, 296, 298 |
| tonic muscles | 64 |
| toning | 19-23, 254-256 |
| trapezius muscle | 57, 61, 248-249, 285 |
| triceps brachii muscle | 48, 285-286 |
| triceps surae muscle | 78, 286-287 |
| ulnar deviation | 32 |
| ulnaris muscle | 29, 44-45 |
| vastus muscles | 278 |
| venous flow | 14 |
| wall | 47-49, 53-54, 71-72, 77-78 |
| warming up | 24-26, 88-89, 230 |
|     brass | 209-214, 218-223 |
|     harp | 166-171 |
|     keyboard | 192-196, 200-205 |
|     percussion | 175-179, 183-188 |
|     strings | 132-136, 140-147, 149-153, 157-162 |
|     winds | 96-101, 106-111, 114-119, 123-128 |
| wind instruments, front | 96-114 |
|     cooling down | 101-105 |
|     warming up | 96-101 |
| wind instruments, lateral | 123-140 |
|     cooling down | 128-131 |
|     warming up | 123-128 |
| wind instruments, side | 114-131 |
|     cooling down | 119-122 |
|     warming up | 114-119 |
| wind instruments, small, front | 106-122 |
|     cooling down | 111-113 |
|     warming up | 106-111 |
| wrists | 25, 29, 31-33, 38-43, 49, 59, 123, 247 |
| zygomaticus major muscle | 273, 287 |

# AUTHORS

## JAUME ROSSET I LLOBET

Dr. Jaume Rosset i Llobet is the founder and medical director of the Institute of Art, Medicine & Physiology (Institut de l'Art, Medicina & Fisiologia www.institutart.com) in Terrassa (Barcelona). He received his bachelor's degree in medicine from the Autonomous University of Barcelona and his Doctorate of Medicine and Surgery (PhD) from the University of Barcelona. Dr. Rosset specializes in medicine for physical education and sports as well as orthopedic surgery and traumatology. He also completed a postgraduate degree in scientific communication. Dr. Rosset is the founder and director of the Medico-Surgical Unit of Art (Unitat Medicoquirúrgica de l'Art) at the General Hospital in Manresa (Barcelona), the first arts medicine unit in a Spanish public hospital. He is also the director of the Foundation for Science and Art (Fundació Ciència i Art www.fcart.org). The recipient of the Professional Excellence Award from the Catalan Medical Association, Dr. Rosset also writes about performing arts medicine for several scientific and educational publications.

## SÍLVIA FÀBREGAS I MOLAS

Silvia Fabregas i Molas is the founder and head of physiotherapy at the Institute of Art, Medicine & Physiology (Institut de l'Art, Medicina & Fisiologia www.institutart.com) in Terrassa (Barcelona). She holds a Diploma in Physiotherapy from the Autonomous University of Barcelona's Gimbernat School. Since its inception, Ms. Fabregas has been a member of the Medical-Surgical of Art unit in the General Hospital in Manresa (Barcelona). As an expert in sports physiotherapy, she has extensive training in the Mezieres, Feldenkrais, and TRAL (Locomotor System Rebalancing Therapy) methods. Ms. Fabregas also has a master's degree in Neuro Linguistic Programming and is responsible for and coordinates the musician's dystonia neurorehabilitation program.

www.ingramcontent.com/pod-product-compliance
Lightning Source LLC
Chambersburg PA
CBHW022036290426
44109CB00014B/872